The Personal
and
the Political

The Personal
and
the Political

Women's Activism in Response to the
Breast Cancer and AIDS Epidemics

Ulrike Boehmer

State University of New York Press

Published by
State University of New York Press, Albany

For information, address State University of New York Press,
State University Plaza, Albany, N.Y., 12246

Production by Michael Haggett
Marketing by Anne M. Valentine

Library of Congress Cataloging-in-Publication Data

Boehmer, Ulrike, 1959–
     The personal and the political : women's activism in response to
the breast cancer and AIDS epidemics / Ulrike Boehmer.
          p.   cm.
     Includes bibliographical references and index.
     ISBN 0-7914-4549-6 (hardcover : alk. paper). — ISBN 0-7914-4550-X
(pbk. : alk. paper)
     1. Breast—Cancer—Political aspects—United States.   2. AIDS
(Disease)—Political aspects—United States.   3. Women political
activists—United States.   I. Title.
RC280.B8B62   2000
362.1'969792'0082—dc21   99-41118
                                                                                      CIP

10 9 8 7 6 5 4 3 2 1

*This book is dedicated
to Dorsey Bushnell.*

Contents

Acknowledgments

Writing a book is mostly an isolating task, in that it requires one to significantly withdraw from friends, people in general, and the very aspect of life that one set out to study. Nevertheless, in hindsight, it is clear that this book would have never been possible without the many people who helped me through the process and whose support made the isolation and the difficulty of the task bearable. I acknowledge those who have contributed to this book in various ways. The foundation for this book is my dissertation work at Boston College. Therefore, I thank the members of my dissertation committee for their feedback and guidance, in particular, William A. Gamson, for his challenging questions that ultimately shaped this project. I also am especially grateful to John B. Williamson, who, over the years, has become a mentor. He generously shared with me his expertise for this project, cooperated with me on many others, and always provided me with valuable career advice. A very special thank-you goes to my dissertation "buddy" and friend Cassie Schwerner, who read my drafts and discussed and scrutinized all of my arguments and ideas. Our exchange of ideas and dissertation materials and mutual support has been the most positive experience of combining the political with the personal and our work with fun.

While a graduate student at Boston College, I also received a lot of intellectual encouragement and support from my peers, including members of the Boston College Media Research and Action Project (MRAP) and members of my dissertation support group. Thanks also to my colleagues at Boston University and the Center for Health Quality, Outcomes, and Economic Research, who listened to me while I produced the final manuscript. Further, the economic support I received at various points allowed me to concentrate fully on writing. Boston College awarded me with a dissertation fellowship, and I received additional financial support from my parents, who, despite all of our differences, have always wanted to help me succeed.

Throughout this project, I have been supported by many friends, my family, and my extended family. I especially thank Joan Vasconcellos and James Vela-McConnell, who shared my graduate student years and who still take an interest in my work. Thanks too to Robert Humphreville for being such a wild friend, and to Costa Pappas, who first introduced me to ACT UP (AIDS Coalition to Unleash Power) and whose memory was an inspiration for this work. My gratitude to Jamy Faust, who encouraged and still encourages me to find pleasure in my work. Also thanks to Andrea Dazzi and all of the members of her energy healing courses, who helped me stay grounded. I am indebted to my extended family in Europe for always reminding me of my roots, of where I am coming from, and for believing that I could do it: Melitta Blagi, Margarethe Wenninger, Dorsey Bushnell, Cornelia Uhlenhaut, Christine Bendel, Wilma Peters, and Chou-Chou. Finally, my thanks to Angela Radan for bringing love, joy, and laughter into my life.

UB
Cambridge, Massachusetts
May 1999

Introduction

The differences between AIDS activism and breast cancer activism became my constant companions during the process of writing this book. I lived in constant tension between these two movements. Most often I experienced these two activist environments as two different worlds. Clearly, my race—white—and my class background—middle class—were well represented in both worlds. I got into the habit of always asking myself how a particular conference or rally would differ if the other health movement had organized it. When I was attending an AIDS-related conference, for example, I often bonded with other gays or lesbians during lunch. However, I noticed that these luncheons generated garbage bags filled with plastic trays, plastic cups, and so forth. This would either not have happened at all or would not have remained unchallenged during a conference that focused on making a link between cancer and the environment.

I attended breast cancer rallies and AIDS walks in Boston. These events, held annually in early summer, are scheduled two weeks apart from each other. My mother was supportive of my being at the breast cancer rally. Breast cancer is a terrible disease, she said. When I talked to her two weeks later to let her know that I was participating in the AIDS walk, I was met with an all too familiar silence that I have learned throughout the years to decode as, "Don't tell me anything about your queer life style; I am working hard on forgetting that part of you." In my mother's eyes, going to the AIDS walk was interchangeable with telling her about going to Gay Pride. My mother, however, is certainly not the only one whose attitudes toward AIDS are entrenched in homophobia and whose reactions to my involvement with breast cancer are much more positive.

Almost everyone I know, myself included, has quite different reactions to breast cancer activism than to AIDS activism. For instance, when I let someone know that I am experiencing a time conflict because I am going to a cancer meeting, I have been asked sometimes directly, "Uli, do you have cancer?" Sometimes people went through the effort of investigating behind my back if I had cancer by asking someone who is close to me and ought to know. Not a single person ever asked me or interrogated my friends if I were HIV-positive when I said I was going to an AIDS event. I spent a great deal of time trying to understand these different reactions, because it seemed to me that the answers to the general question I was posing, why women become active in one or the other movement, were closely related to the difference between reactions, to breast cancer and AIDS.

What does the difference mean? My guess is that the immediate and unquestioned acceptance of my attending AIDS meetings is grounded in others' perceptions of AIDS as a political issue. In addition, those who know I am a lesbian seem to find my attendance of AIDS meetings almost self-explanatory. A similar justification between breast cancer and my being a lesbian was never made by others. It seems that not even being a woman can explain my attendance at breast cancer meetings; the overriding fact is that I do not have cancer. It was never assumed that anyone could attend such meetings for political reasons.

My personal experiences concerning the general perceptions of AIDS and breast cancer seem to reflect how differently these two issues are perceived. For the breast cancer and AIDS walks that I mentioned earlier, the difference was also expressed in numbers. In 1995, the breast cancer march and rally was held on a sunny Sunday in late May. Approximately 2,000, mostly white women, attended the event. In contrast, 30,000 attended the tenth annual AIDS pledge walk in Boston that took place two weeks later on a dreary Sunday at the beginning of June that year. The people who had collected pledges for walking 10 kilometers came from different backgrounds: straight and gay, young and old, from families, and of many different races and ethnicities. After the event, the diversity of the walkers was also mirrored by the speakers who addressed the audience and congratulated everybody about the success of raising millions of dollars for various AIDS organizations. After the AIDS walk, some of the speakers spoke to me, a white middle-class lesbian concerned about the future of the gay and lesbian community and the funding of AIDS organizations. In comparison, at the breast cancer rally, speakers talked about the experiences of their treatments. While this made me look at these women and marvel about their courage, it also frightened me. I was terrified about the future of my friends who have cancer, and it scared me to think that I might have a cancer diagnosis one day and might have to undergo similar treatments. While most of these speakers were white and middle class, what separated me from them was not their cancer diagnosis but rather their accounts of loving and supportive husbands and their concern for their children. If I were ever in the situation of having cancer treatments, I would have to not only decide on which treatment but ponder whether I would receive the same kind of care and attention as these straight women if it were known that I was a lesbian. Even though I knew that some of the speakers were lesbians, none of them either shared the experience of a lesbian who underwent treatment or addressed specific lesbian concerns, such as negotiating health care in a homophobic environment.

In my personal life, the distinction between cancer and AIDS is expressed through the reactions of my friends. Whereas I have to attend the annual breast cancer rally alone, many of my friends volunteer to come with me to the more time-intensive, longer, and more strenuous annual AIDS walk. I am familiar with this difference in response because it was not long ago that I myself perceived the breast cancer movement as being quite different from the AIDS movement. I attended AIDS walks but not cancer rallies.

I have always been aware of the AIDS movement. The first time I heard about AIDS, my interest was immediately triggered. In 1982, a friend of mine, Dorsey, who was studying to be a nurse, told me about gay and lesbian health professionals who got together to compile information on a new disease called "gay cancer" that was occurring in gay men. Intuitively, it made sense to me that gays and lesbians should get together to educate each other about the disease. It did not have to be exchanged verbally—we assumed that the dominant institutions in society were run by people who perpetuate heterosexism and therefore would not care if we live or die. In order to survive, we had to look out for ourselves by taking care of each other. From that time on, I kept abreast of any new developments within AIDS activism. At this time, I did not consider myself to be interested in health issues, and I did not perceive AIDS predominantly as a health issue. It was not the disease component of AIDS that held my attention; from the beginning, I perceived AIDS as a gay and lesbian rights issue, and that was why it affected me long before I ever knew someone who had been infected.

Maybe that is why I was much more reserved when I read about the formation of a breast cancer movement in the early 1990s. It piqued my interest because it was the emergence of a movement. At that time, I perceived breast cancer activism as being a much more disease-focused movement. I got a lot of the information about breast cancer, at the time, through an AIDS perspective. I often received the information in the context of moving loosely in the arena of AIDS activism. It was discussed there, because AIDS activists wondered what the breast cancer movement would mean for the future of AIDS funding.

My detached observer status to the emerging breast cancer movement was terminated when Dorsey was diagnosed with breast cancer in the spring of 1992—ten years after she informed me about the "gay cancer." I began reading the available information about breast cancer differently. I wanted to find out in more detail about the activities and goals of this new movement. Actually, Dorsey was not the first woman I ever knew with breast cancer, but she was the first with cancer to whom I was close and who was from my own age group. Earlier, some of my parents' friends whom I had known since early childhood had been diagnosed with breast cancer and had died of it. Despite knowing these women personally for 30 years or more, I perceived their diagnoses as being no different from any other health problem that people might encounter in their lifetime. Even attending Audre Lorde's readings, which she gave during her extended stays in West Berlin, where she was receiving alternative cancer treatments, did not cause a reaction similar to my initial one when I had heard about AIDS. I reacted much more strongly to Audre Lorde's other identities—being an African-American lesbian who created awareness about and eventually an organization of African-German women.

In 1993, my perception of breast cancer from being a disease to being a political issue that affected me was made clear when I read the headline in the *Boston Globe*, "Breast Cancer Risk in Lesbians Put at 1 in 3."[1] This news report got my attention. My interest was piqued enough to expand my dissertation that I had always intended to be a study on women in the AIDS movement into a comparative analysis of women in the breast cancer movement and the AIDS movement.

These personal revelations indicate how long it took me to become interested in breast cancer activism. Only after I had opened up to political awareness about both health concerns could I also experience their similarities. One basic similarity was that women's medical treatment lagged behind men's, and that both diseases were taking an incredible toll on human lives. For instance, I was attempting to interview two women, one in AIDS activism and one in breast cancer activism, for months. I was constantly being told, "When I feel better, I will do it." Unfortunately, I was eventually informed about their deaths. Thus the words of all of the women I did get a chance to interview have been incredibly valuable. I have done my best to respect these women's words by letting them speak for themselves as much as my role as researcher and author has allowed me to. I owe the interviewed women who gave me their time and shared their thoughts much more than being provided with data for this book. Most of all, I am grateful to them because they have taught me in personal and political ways that have changed me. I have learned how everyone's political awakening is different and that it happens at different times in the course of people's lives. One of the deeply personal lessons I have learned is to accept that life, and every aspect of it, is always uncertain and temporary.

CHAPTER 1

A History of AIDS
and Breast Cancer Activism

A synopsis of the history of AIDS and breast cancer activism involves focusing on three different eras. Prior to the 1980s, organizational responses to cancer emerged, many of which are still in existence today. The second era encompasses the 1980s, during which time grassroots organizing occurred in response to the suddenly emerging new disease, AIDS. Finally, the third era begins roughly with the late 1980s and early 1990s. During this time, AIDS organizations became firmly established and grassroots breast cancer activism emerged.

What follows is a brief summary of various events that preceded the cancer and AIDS activism of today. Several comprehensive histories of cancer, AIDS, and the women's health movement have been written by others. I will draw heavily on these works. My selection of historic context attempts to provide the reader with what I consider essential information for a discussion of today's women cancer and AIDS activists who are the focus of this book.

Breast cancer organizing in the pre-AIDS era

Breast cancer has existed as a disease for a long time. During this time, there have been various organizational responses to the disease that preceded the breast cancer activism of the 1990s. It is beyond the scope of this book to reiterate the various phases of organizational responses to cancer, yet for an understanding of today's organizing around cancer it is essential to know that women have been central in responding to cancer in earlier times.

James Patterson chronicles cancer within American culture. He writes, "Nineteen thirteen marked the completion of the first wave of organization and philanthropy in the field of cancer research."[1] During that year, the American Society for the Control of Cancer was formed. This voluntary health organization did not engage in research directly. Rather, the organization compiled statistics and educated the public about cancer, its early warning signs, and detection. This precursor of the American Cancer Society was founded by a woman, Mrs. Robert G. Mead. Its founding was publicized by the *New York Times* as "Rich Women Begin a War on Cancer."[2] This voluntary organization, the American Society for the Control of Cancer, continued for many years through ups and downs and experienced a change in its leadership from a medical elite towards more business-minded people, who in 1946 renamed the organization the American Cancer Society.

Patterson mentions Mary Lasker as being a key figure in transforming the more modest American Society for the Control of Cancer into the financial giant, the American Cancer Society (hereafter, ACS). Ironically, "Lasker was the wife of advertising tycoon Albert Lasker, who pioneered a campaign urging women to smoke, using the slogan, 'Reach for a Lucky Instead of a Sweet.' "[3] Despite women's influential role in the formation and continuation of the ACS, the organization was criticized, beginning in the 1970s, for its gender politics. The ACS is a male-dominated agency in the sense that men hold the powerful positions, although a majority of women donate their time and volunteer for the organization and its programs, such as "Reach to Recovery." Terese Lasser, a woman who had undergone a mastectomy herself, began the Reach to Recovery program in 1952. This program was later adopted by the American Cancer Society.[4]

Today, the American Cancer Society is considered a prominent part of the "cancer establishment"[5] and is much criticized by cancer activists. The ACS grew into a multimillion dollar project; it is the largest private charity organization in the United States.[6] and calls more than 2 million volunteers its real strength.[7]

Criticism of the cancer establishment was voiced in the late 1970s and early 1980s.[8] Among the criticism was that the cancer establishment is a high-powered, special-interest lobby that held a lot of financial power and whose members made their living off of cancer.[9] The ACS was specifically criticized for its constantly cheerful attitude it puts forward, despite a continuous increase in cancer. In addition to knowing about how the best known bureaucratic cancer organization (ACS) came into existence, and how women made an important contribution to cancer organizing, I shift the attention to another early precursor of cancer in the public arena.

During the early 1970s, despite anti-establishment feelings that had been triggered by the Vietnam War, the confidence and expertise of medical experts was still unchallenged. Even though Patterson acknowledges that many expressed anger or doubts and resentment toward cancer and its cure, he concludes that, "What they shared was a mood, not a passion for organization or coalition. For all these reasons no united movement against the anticancer alliance developed in the 1960s."[10] He points to the late 1960s as a time when there was extraordinary pressure on the federal government to lead a war on cancer. Mary Lasker, who transformed the ACS, was instrumental in leading a campaign that demanded more money for cancer research. One of the arguments was, "The war in Vietnam . . . had killed some 41,000 Americans in four years, whereas cancer had killed 320,000 in one."[11] The Lasker alliance, which pushed for more cancer funding, put its confidence into the government, assuming that more spending on research would eventually bring the cancer cure. Further, a redistribution of government spending from defense to cancer was demanded. This is the same argument that cancer activists voiced in the mid-1990s.

The advocates for cancer funding eventually succeeded. One of the reasons for their success is that cancer is an issue that can find a broad base of supporters and unite liberals and conservatives alike. Patterson quotes one contemporary observer, who commented that, "To oppose big spending against cancer was . . . to oppose Mom, apple pie, and the flag."[12] The success of cancer spending advocacy was finalized when President Nixon signed the National Cancer Act in 1971. This bill was seen as the beginning of the "war on cancer." It secured more funding for the National Cancer Institute (NCI) and gave the agency special status among the institutes of the National Institutes of Health (NIH). Further, attached to this legislative bill were expectations that the United States should become the first nation to discover a cancer cure. When the success was elusive and no cure was found, the war on cancer eventually had stalled by the end of the 1970s.

Of further interest for an understanding of cancer activism of the 1990s is the wave of "coming out" or "going public" by well-known women who had been diagnosed with breast cancer in the mid-1970s. The media paid attention to prominent women who underwent breast cancer surgery: "Marvella Bayh, wife of Indiana Senator Birch Bayh, the actress Shirley Temple Black, and [within a month of each other in 1974] Betty Ford and Happy Rockefeller."[13] One of the immediate results of the well-publicized mastectomies that the president's and the vice president's wives underwent was that the number of diagnosed breast cancers increased, presumably because more women themselves had been screened.[14] Of special interest was the media's framing of the cancer experience of the First and Second Ladies. Newspaper reports were filled with assurances that Betty Ford and Happy Rockefeller were accepting of their surgeries, had their loving husbands at their sides, were in excellent spirits, and had speedy recoveries. Regaining complete mobility after surgery was visually symbolized by a picture of Betty Ford tossing a football a few days after her mastectomy.[15] Betty Ford was also quoted as advising other women, "Once it's done, put it behind you and go on with your life."[16]

Rose Kushner[17] is considered one breast cancer activist of the pre-AIDS era, beginning in the late 1970s and lasting until the mid-1980s. Her feminist stand differs gravely from the framing of the First and Second Ladies' surgeries. Ford and Rockefeller underwent Halsted radical mastectomies[18] because this method had been chosen as appropriate by their husbands after consultation with the doctors. Moreover, Rockefeller underwent a second mastectomy a few weeks after her first one because she had been diagnosed with carcinoma in situ[19] in her other breast.

> Vice President Rockefeller told the millions in his radio and TV audience that he had withheld this information from his wife after the first operation because of her emotional state. . . . Finally, in the middle of November, Happy Rockefeller was informed of her fate. The second breast was removed as the men around her had decided.[20]

Contrary to such paternalistic behavior and portrayal of women's breast cancer surgeries, Rose Kushner and other women have taken a feminist position. Their approach to breast cancer had been influenced by the second wave of women's liberation in the late 1960s and early 1970s and by the emergence of the women's health movement. At the core of the women's health movement was the belief that women must have ultimate control over their bodies. This has been put forward by the Boston Women's Health Book Collective, which, since 1972, has published collaboratively their groundbreaking work *Our Bodies, Ourselves.* Further, other national organizations such as the Women's Health Network emerged, along with many local self-help groups all over the country.

In 1981, Byllye Avery founded with others the National Black Women's Health Project, which counts many local self-help groups, plus groups in Kenya, Barbados, and Belize, among its members. This umbrella organization is conceptualized around an understanding of health from the perspective of black women. This perspective either is completely ignored by health and medical literature or neglects to put health into a format that makes sense to black women.[21] Other health organizations by women of color have emerged as well, for example, the National Latina Health Organization, which was formed to raise Latina consciousness, and the Native Women Reproductive Rights Coalition, which promotes productive rights for Native American women.[22]

Media attention to breast cancer diagnoses of prominent women, the emerging women's health movement, and the needs of many women who had undergone breast cancer surgery led to the formation of breast cancer survivor groups in the late 1970s. These groups functioned as important resources and support systems for women who were living with this disease.[23] Such patient-driven self-help and support groups are frequently closely aligned with hospitals and built the dominant breast cancer organizational type of the pre-AIDS era. Many of these support groups were organized under the National Alliance of Breast Cancer Organizations (NABCO), a national umbrella organization founded in 1986 by Kushner and other women. This nonprofit organization defines itself as a resource for medical, surgical, psychological, and legal progress regarding breast cancer in the United States.[24] NABCO has linked pre-AIDS times with the advocacy-driven post-AIDS[25] breast cancer activism of the 1990s, and it is among the primary organizers of the National Breast Cancer Coalition (NBCC), a national advocacy organization founded in 1991.[26]

A second connection between pre-AIDS times and the 1990s has occurred with regard to patient-driven self-help groups. These groups, closely aligned with hospitals, still exist today. They continue to give valuable support and information to women who share in the experience of a cancer diagnosis. However, several of the grassroots breast cancer activism groups of the 1990s, on whose members this book focuses, expanded on the former self-help groups by offering support within the context of political advocacy.

Third, an early pioneer who carried breast cancer organizing into the 1990s was Audre Lorde. She published *The Cancer Journals* in 1980, and her writings continued to raise awareness about cancer until she died of breast cancer in 1992. Lorde outlined a political response to breast cancer and demanded political action on breast cancer long before grassroots cancer groups organized to do so in the late 1980s and 1990s. Moreover, *The Cancer Journals* contained Lorde's speech on "The Transformation of Silence into Language and Action," which she had delivered in 1977.[27] In it she was voicing statements about silence and cancer, years before the famous "Silence = Death" slogan of the AIDS movement appeared in 1986.[28]

AIDS organizing

This brief history of organizational responses to the AIDS crisis gives the reader some background facts that are helpful in understanding *women's* AIDS activism of today. My focus on women's activism may differ from readers' preexisting knowledge about the AIDS epidemic and AIDS activism, which is most likely generated by the highly publicized AIDS history that commonly stems from a male perspective. Even though the majority of AIDS organizations of both the beginning years and today are gender-mixed ones, I do not present women's activism as a comparison to men's activism.[29]

The World Health Organization (WHO) has divided the AIDS epidemic's history into three periods: "the silent period (ca. 1970–1981), the initial discovery (1981–1985), and worldwide mobilization (1985–1988)."[30] This division of the epidemic's history supports an important argument that a number of authors have made. It is the argument that an adequate organizational response by the public health officials to the AIDS crisis in the United States was delayed because of society's and the health organizations' homophobia.[31]

Overall, the public health officials' response was one of neglect. Their lack of action lasted until the mid-1980s, when the perception of AIDS shifted from being a "gay disease" to being a threat for the "general population" or "heterosexual community."[32] Early on, this caused the gay and lesbian community to respond to the epidemic by pulling together their own resources. Gay and lesbian community-based AIDS organizations were in place by 1985 and had achieved hegemony when public health officials finally responded.[33] AIDS service organizations emerged first in the three epicenters of the HIV epidemic (New York, Los Angeles, and San Francisco). They shaped organizational styles that were picked up by second-tier cities such as Boston, Chicago, Washington, Atlanta, and Houston.[34]

Further, early AIDS organizers oriented themselves toward other health-related organizations, the foremost being cancer organizations, such as the ACS.[35] That early AIDS organizers envisioned an AIDS organization similar to the ACS is one of many examples that shows how organizational responses to these two diseases are interrelated.

At first, gay community-based AIDS service organizations started with an uncritical view of modern medicine, one that expected to find a cure for AIDS. Such an approach to modern medicine was soon replaced, however, by a critical political analysis of medicine and health care. Dennis Altman credits the lesbians who were active in AIDS organizations with having caused this shift in thinking:

> The growth of AIDS organizations has not meant a corresponding growth in analysis of medicine and health as a social and political issue. Where such analysis has occurred, it was often due to the work of lesbians, many of whom had already been active in feminist health groups.[36]

Altman characterizes the organizational response of the gay and lesbian community as having a historical parallel to the women's movement of the 1970s. AIDS organizing of the 1980s became the most visible effort of the gay and lesbian community, similar to women's health concerns (such as reproductive rights), which had often been the most visible feminist activities of the women's movement in the 1970s. Nevertheless, Altman concludes that while AIDS had brought gay men and lesbians closer together, it also clearly highlighted the differences between the two. Gay male issues took center stage, but lesbians' health concerns remained unacknowledged.

The history of organizational responses to AIDS is narrated differently with regard to women's contribution depending on the author covering the period. The best-known chronicle of the AIDS epidemic—*And the Band Played On*—has been criticized for its many shortcomings.[37] I like to emphasize that Shilts' lack of acknowledgment of women's activism is among his serious shortcomings. Concerning the omission of women from the history of AIDS organizing, Judy Macks and Caitlin Ryan write the following:

> The pioneering contributions of lesbians have been lost or obscured as the written and oral history of AIDS has been reported in both the general and gay press. The involvement of lesbians in the formation of community-based AIDS organizations as direct service providers, fundraisers, community organizers, educators and activists has rarely been acknowledged. Yet that does not make our varied contributions any less real, historic or vital.[38]

The motivations for lesbians and straight women to be part of the AIDS movement are discussed in chapter 4. Cindy Patton's assessment of women's activism is that by the mid-1980s, white middle-class straight women had joined the AIDS service organizations as volunteers.[39]

Around that time, other changes occurred within AIDS organizations. Following the gay and lesbian community that had responded to AIDS first, other communities acted according to their cultural framework. Within communities of color, AIDS was first added as yet one more issue for already existing multiservice organizations that had always been catering to the Haitian, African-American, or Latino communities. Only later did single-issue AIDS organizations emerge in communities of color as well as AIDS organizations that targeted women specifically. The gay community-based AIDS service organizations adjusted to the changing face of the epidemic by expanding their services and catering to women and communities of color.[40] Beth Schneider discusses the mobilization of affected peoples and communities:

> Shaw (1988) documents in her analysis of community organizing efforts, the course of mobilization for women and ethnic minority communities necessarily differs from that of the gay community given aggregate differences in wealth and political power and, hence, in the ability to marshal resources. . . . In most large cities, there has been a proliferation of AIDS organizations as the lack of governmental funds and municipal services placed responsibility for the crisis squarely on the shoulders of the communities most affected. The emergence of a private sector of nonprofit organizations devoted to AIDS, reliant on volunteers from the lesbian/gay community, partially masked the failure of, or virtual lack of, health care delivery.[41]

One seldom acknowledged arena is the responses by prostitutes who were active in self-empowerment and prostitute rights organizations. These women acted as AIDS peer educators for other prostitutes. Similarly, a less publicized response was AIDS education projects that emerged in prisons.[42] AIDS also formed many new communities such as the People Living with AIDS movement (PLWA), which was launched in 1983.[43]

The founding of ACT UP (AIDS Coalition to Unleash Power) in New York in March 1987 marked a revolutionary shift in AIDS organizing and activism. ACT UP chapters were soon mushrooming all over the country and spread as far as the major cities of Western Europe, South America, Australia, and South Africa. This "diverse, nonpartisan group of individuals united in anger and committed to direct action to end the AIDS crisis"[44] consisted predominantly of white gay men and lesbians. ACT UP effectively used the media and engaged in many actions of civil disobedience that targeted institutions such as government agencies, pharmaceutical industries, and anyone who was perceived as harmful to their declared goal—ending the AIDS crisis. ACT UP's actions became widely known through their presence in the media. The organization came to symbolize AIDS activism of the late 1980s and early 1990s. ACT UP shifted the strategy from the political activism of the early years and organizing around AIDS to a direct and visible approach. ACT UP was not, however, the beginning of AIDS activism.

ACT UP has been sometimes perceived as an organization of angry gay white men who came together motivated by self-interest. That perception is erroneous. Perceiving ACT UP in such a way denies the importance and participation of women. Moreover, ACT UP's actions were instrumental in publicizing the discrimination that women and people of color with AIDS endured. Therefore, the organization has to be credited with being at least partially successful in eliminating the discrimination that these groups suffered. As a matter of fact, the women's caucus of ACT UP brought a feminist analysis to the AIDS crisis; that is, the women in ACT UP publicized the ways in which women with AIDS have been scapegoated and framed as carriers of the disease. Women were often blamed for giving AIDS to their children. Prior to ACT UP's highly publicized actions, women and people of color had frequently been excluded from experimental drug trials. Finally, ACT UP's women fought the CDC (Centers for Disease Control) to change its AIDS definition to include the women-specific HIV/AIDS-related symptoms.[45]

The women AIDS activists interviewed for this book come from any of these organizational responses to AIDS that reach from gay community-based to community of color-based, women-only AIDS organizations, or to advocacy-only AIDS organizations.

Breast cancer activism in the post-AIDS era

The zeitgeist in the post-AIDS era has both enabled and constrained grassroots organizational responses to breast cancer. AIDS has been an enabler for the grassroots breast cancer movement in the 1990s, because AIDS activism has served as a model for organizing around a disease.[46] On the other hand, there is also ample evidence that these two diseases have been pitted against each other by politicians who were deciding about the distribution of resources.

The general perception that AIDS organizing had been tremendously successful in changing AIDS policies set off a spark in women and triggered organizing and activism around breast cancer. While AIDS organizing has been widely acknowledged as the model for breast cancer activism, there exists a second legacy upon which the breast cancer movement draws—the women's health movement. Organizational responses around women's health are one organizational background for many women who have entered AIDS activism. Hence, AIDS and breast cancer organizing weaves together different organizational resources. Women within AIDS were able to draw on their experiences in the women's movement and the women's health movement in particular, while women in the breast cancer movement were able to draw on AIDS organizing as a model. Since the breast cancer movement of today draws on both AIDS and the women's health movement, it has created a new organizational hybrid.[47]

Activist grassroots breast cancer organizations expanded in the late 1980s in various parts of the country. Some examples of early cancer activist organizations follow: In Berkeley, California, Jackie Winnow, a lesbian and an AIDS activist who had been diagnosed with breast cancer in 1985 and metastatic disease in 1988, founded the Women's Cancer Resource Center. In 1989, the Boston-based feminist Susan Shapiro, who had breast cancer, published an article in the feminist newspaper *Sojourner* entitled "Cancer As a Feminist Issue," in which she called on women to attend a meeting. Women followed her call, and from this meeting emerged the Women's Community Cancer Project of Cambridge, Massachusetts. A different organizational type, the Mary-Helen Mautner Project for Lesbians with Cancer, opened its doors in Washington, D.C., in January 1990. This project was founded by Susan Hester, after Mautner, her partner, died of breast cancer in her early forties. The Mautner project is modeled after the AIDS buddy system,[48] and its main focus is on providing services to lesbians with cancer. Advocacy for lesbians is an additional part to the main mission of caring for lesbians with cancer. In July 1990, Eleanor Pred, a veteran of the civil rights and antiwar movement of the 1960s, founded Breast Cancer Action in San Francisco, consciously modeling the organization after AIDS activist organizations.[49]

These organizations largely exemplify the differences among the existing grassroots activist cancer organizations of today. While all of these organizations are political organizations based on the understanding that cancer is a political issue that has to be tackled through advocacy, some women's organizations focus on all cancers, others on just breast cancer, and some exclusively on lesbians and cancer. Further, these different advocacy organizations provide varying degrees of direct services for women and lesbians with cancer. Some of today's organizations are only dedicated to advocacy, some combine advocacy with a support group, and some function as a direct service agency combined with activism.

These activist organizations began to merge into national organizations in the early 1990s. In April 1991, the National Coalition of Feminist and Lesbian Cancer Projects was formed after a panel discussion at the National Lesbian Conference in Atlanta.[50] In May 1991, the National Breast Cancer Coalition was formed in Washington, D.C.[51] The political goals of these activist organizations and their national umbrella organizations as well as the goals of AIDS activism are discussed next.

Political goals of the movements

There are certain differences and similarities in terms of the political goals of the two movements. At the beginning, emerging AIDS organizations provided services for people with AIDS and pressed for research dollars both to find a cure and through education to prevent the further spread of the disease. Overall, these broad goals were not unlike those of the cancer movement. With cancer, similar goals were put forward: prevention of cancer by finding its causes and, sometimes, access for women with cancer. Organizations that emphasized direct services are replicating what the AIDS movement had put forth as a model. Predominantly service-oriented organizations are lesbian organizations such as the Mautner Project in Washington, D.C., and the Lesbian Community Project in Chicago. But the biggest effort of the breast cancer movement has been to raise dollars for research on the causes of breast cancer—research that investigates the link between cancer and the environment.

The issue of prevention marks a difference between the two movements. After all, AIDS is a preventable disease, whereas cancer is not, since its causes are still unknown. While the AIDS movement puts most of its pressure on finding a vaccine, or at least on developing drugs that prolong life for people with HIV/AIDS, the cancer movement relies primarily on basic scientific research to find the causes of cancer. While one of the biggest accomplishments of the AIDS movement has been to revolutionize how drug trials are administered and how new drugs are approved by the FDA, the cancer movement's revolutionary aspect has been to bring attention to the disease and the toll it takes on women's lives. Contrary to the AIDS movement, the cancer movement seeks to decrease research that focuses on drug-related issues, such as specifying amounts of chemotherapy and the length of time a woman undergoes chemotherapy, and instead to shift the research focus to the environmental causes of cancer. With cancer, drug-focused research has for many years been dominant and has traditionally been done by and in cooperation with pharmaceutical industries. The cancer activists of today demand instead that research ought to focus foremost on prevention—especially as cancer activists point out, since the treatments for cancer have not changed in the last fifty years. They have included surgery, radiation, and chemotherapy, or, as many refer to them, "slash, burn, and poison."

From this focus, a certain direction and political strategy emerge concerning the implementation of goals. There is no single strategy that summarizes the politics of all grassroots cancer organizations. The decision of which goal to implement (i.e., access, direct service, education, advocacy, cure, or prevention) differs from one organization to the next. While the strategy of the National Breast Cancer Coalition is heavily influenced by an understanding that breast cancer is a bipartisan issue, other local grassroots cancer organizations take a more radical stand.

Some of these more radical cancer organizations push most heavily for prevention by focusing on the environmental causes of breast cancer. They thereby draw a line between grassroots cancer organizations, on the one side, and the cancer establishment (e.g., the ACS), pharmaceutical industries, and large corporations that manufacture cancer-causing products or pollute the environment, on the other side.[52] By dividing the arena in this way, these environmentally concerned and motivated cancer organizations seek to build an anti-cancer lobby and turn to various environmental organizations such as Greenpeace for coalition building around the environment.[53]

The broad goals of AIDS organizations and the AIDS movement are similar to the goals of cancer organizations and the cancer movement. For instance, the Women and AIDS Coalition in Washington, D.C., states its mission as follows:

> The Women and AIDS Coalition takes its direction from the women on the front-lines; we are working to open doors so that more women will feel for the first time as though they have access to and representation in processes which will profoundly affect their lives. The participants work together to bring women's perspectives to the AIDS policy arena and to ensure that women's concerns are not neglected in federal legislative and executive branch HIV/AIDS policy. . . . We work with other NORA [National Organizations Responding to AIDS] Task Forces to incorporate women's needs in prevention, care and treatment, and research priorities for federal funding.[54]

However, coalition building and working relationships within the AIDS arena are distinctly different from coalition building and working relationships within cancer.

Whereas more radical cancer activists argue against a unity with the cancer establishment and have chosen to build coalitions outside of the establishment, coalitions and relationships in the AIDS arena started from an opposite vantage point. Since its emergence, AIDS had been strongly linked to homophobia, and because of this connection, gays and lesbians were confronted with homophobic government officials and civic powers. Therefore, early AIDS activists who were gays and lesbians started as outsiders and sought to influence public policies around HIV/AIDS and to exert pressure for anti-discrimination ordinances for people with HIV/AIDS. Further, one of the greatest successes of the AIDS movement has been that AIDS activists have built working relationships with large pharmaceutical companies and have obtained standing as consumer advocates who are included at the table when new drug applications are investigated.

Cindy Patton argues that a shift from initial grassroots responses by the gay and lesbian community to a more assimilated AIDS service organization structure occurred in the mid-1980s.[55] However, Patton points out that, prior to 1986, the gay and lesbian response to AIDS was framed by empowerment through community self-determination. The search for AIDS services was internal to the gay and lesbian community and independent, because government had historically shown antagonism toward gay men—including personal surveillance. Patton distinguishes this analysis within the gay and lesbian community from an analysis within the African-American community. African Americans were much more inclined to view social problems within their community as an outcome of government discrimination. An empowerment strategy for the African American community is to demand governmental services and access in payment for years of discrimination.

The shift by gay community-based AIDS service organizations to work more closely with the government beginning in the mid-1980s intensified even further toward assimilation through an influential decision that gay AIDS activists made in the mid to late 1980s. To gain more access to resources and to attract more attention to the disease, gay AIDS leaders made a conscious political choice to "de-gay" AIDS.[56] These leaders' rationale for a de-gaying of AIDS was that society's deep-seated homophobia required such a step to remove the stigma of homosexuality from AIDS. The strategy of de-gaying AIDS meant, among others, to build single-issue AIDS organizations, to use nongays as spokespeople, to focus narrowly on AIDS instead of on the underlying themes of racism and homophobia, and to emphasize that AIDS is not a gay disease. In hindsight, this decision of de-gaying AIDS has been acknowledged as being highly problematic, because it realized its short-term gains but in the long term depoliticized AIDS by separating it from its gay and lesbian liberationist roots.[57] Along with the decision to de-gay AIDS, AIDS became de-sexualized when attention shifted from gay male sex to committed gay male relationships. This decision is under revision today by some of the same gay men who were initially influential in the de-gaying of AIDS.[58]

In summary

Within this section, the two health-related movements have been located within their historical political context. The differences and similarities have been discussed and highlighted that have both set the two movements apart from each other and provided similar struggles for each. Further, it is noteworthy how intertwined the two movements are. The AIDS movement benefited from the experiences of feminist and women's health movement activists, while the breast cancer movement of the 1990s used the experiences of AIDS activism and feminist strategies as its roots. With regard to politics, the two movements have started from opposite vantage points. AIDS had been linked to male homosexuality; consequently, AIDS activists began outside of the political arena struggling for influence through a strategy of assimilation and coalition building with straight health officials, government officials, and drug industries. In contrast, breast cancer started as a mainstream issue; therefore, the progressives among cancer activists have pushed against coalition building with a cancer establishment that has neither served them nor represented their interests in the many years of their existence.

CHAPTER 2

Activism and Activists: Definitions and Selection Criteria

In this chapter, I address the specifics that underlie this study. The prevalence of the diseases among women, the perspective chosen, the definition of activism itself, the selection of individual activists who have been interviewed, and the relevance of these choices are all discussed in this chapter.

Who has AIDS and breast cancer?

AIDS and breast cancer represent health crises that affect various segments of the population. However, women at risk for developing breast cancer are different from women at risk for HIV infection. Breast cancer takes a greater toll on the female population than does AIDS.[1] Like any infectious disease, AIDS affects predominantly the disadvantaged within society. The incidence of breast cancer is counter to society's discriminatory practices in that white women are at the highest risk of developing breast cancer (about 1 in 7 women), and higher socioeconomic status is a risk factor of the disease.[2] Breast cancer is less prevalent among African American, Hispanic, Asian, and other non-white women; however, when one controls for age, African-

American women have a higher incidence at an earlier age, and white women tend to have a higher incidence of breast cancer after fifty years of age.[3] African-American women's breast cancer risk is about 1 in 9 women, but they are more likely to die of this disease as compared to white women.[4] This association persists, even after income is controlled.[5] The American Cancer Society (ACS) attributes the difference in mortality between whites and African Americans mainly to late diagnosis.[6] The National Cancer Institute (NCI) found that lack of health insurance is an important predictor of mortality.[7]

The prevalence of breast cancer among lesbians is uncertain, because lesbians are invisibilized in society and women's health studies tend to omit questions about women's sexual orientation, which leads to the current lack of any generalizable data on lesbians. A NCI epidemiologist, Suzanne G. Haynes, publicized in 1993 findings of her study, which showed that lesbians have a 1 in 3 lifetime risk of developing breast cancer, which is about three times the risk of heterosexual women (1 in 8).[8] Haynes performed these calculations using data that had been collected on the lesbian community,[9] and found that lesbians have the following characteristics: they smoke more, they are more likely to use and abuse alcohol, they have a higher body mass index, they give birth less frequently, they obtain fewer screening exams (e.g., Pap smear, breast exam, mammogram), and they have lower rates of self-care (e.g., breast self-exam, doctor visits for pain).[10] Most of these characteristics of self-identified lesbians are risk factors for breast cancer, which explains Haynes' finding of a higher breast cancer risk for lesbians. In 1999, the Institute of Medicine published its report on lesbian health.[11] The groundbreaking report states that lesbians have mostly been overlooked, and it stresses the importance of future studies of lesbian health issues. Among the areas that require attention are health conditions for which lesbians are at risk or tend to be at greater risk compared to heterosexual women.

> In the face of little empirical information, there are numerous beliefs, myths, and misconceptions about the health risks of lesbians that can affect their health outcomes. These beliefs are often shared both by health care providers and by lesbians themselves. Some of these beliefs may be true; others are not. These beliefs include perceptions that lesbians do not need regular Pap tests or routine gynecological care, that they do not contract HIV/AIDS, and that there is an epidemic of breast cancer in the lesbian community.[12]

Initially, HIV/AIDS has been associated with gay men. Proportionally, HIV disease affects more men (of all sexual orientations), but women made up 22 percent of AIDS cases in 1998.[13] Further, from 1985 to 1997, the proportion of AIDS cases in women reported each year increased from 7 percent to 22 percent.[14] Minority women are disproportionately affected. In 1996, 56 percent of female AIDS cases were among African-American women, and 20 percent were among Hispanic women. These women tend to be young and poor and live in disenfranchised inner-city neighborhoods.[15] AIDS is now the third leading cause of death among women ages twenty-five to forty-four and the leading cause of death among African-American women in this age group.[16] The decrease in AIDS deaths due to the new treatments are greater in men than in women (44 percent and 32 percent, respectively).[17] Among women diagnosed with AIDS in 1998, most contracted HIV through heterosexual contact (37 percent).[18] During unprotected heterosexual intercourse, women are more likely to be infected than men.[19] In 1998, the second largest group of HIV in women is related to injection drug use (30 percent).[20] Further, women's exposure category is more frequently other or unidentified risk (31 percent) compared to men (21 percent).[21] Again, data on lesbians and HIV are not available, especially since the Centers for Disease Control (CDC) omits female-to-female transmission as an exposure category of HIV. However, a study is currently underway attempting to explain why women intravenous (IV) drug users who report having sex with women have higher levels of HIV infection compared to other IV drug users.[22] While women whose HIV infections are detected early and who receive appropriate treatment survive as long as infected men, several studies have indicated that women's survival times tend to be shorter due to later detection, less access, or use of health care resources.[23] In summary, there are differences and similarities between AIDS and breast cancer. Among the differences is the fact that women who are at the highest risk for contracting HIV or developing cancer come from opposite socioeconomic and racial backgrounds. However, these two diseases share many similarities. Health care practice, health research, clinical research, and research funding have been shown to be discriminatory due to gender, race, and sexual orientation based biases.[24]

What approach to take?

My perspective takes as a given that the AIDS movement and the breast cancer movement emerged in response to these health crises that have reached epidemic proportions in the United States. I use the words "AIDS and cancer movement" interchangeably with "AIDS and cancer activism" throughout this book. These terms capture the societal response of individuals whom I describe as the group of AIDS or cancer activists and from whom I selected my interviewees. My focus for this study is on the women within these two movements. Therefore, I am not focusing on the origin or the development of these two movements and the societal conditions that have been enabling or constraining.

The AIDS and breast cancer movements have been studied from a variety of perspectives, including certain facts and people, while excluding others. The questions asked and answers sought are determined by the particular perspective that one takes. My particular view is rooted in social movement and feminist theory and scholarship. Social movement theorists frequently focus on macro issues that seek to determine the success of movements. Often movement theorists emphasize the structural constraints of and opportunities available to movements. While this perspective on protest movements and their opposition connects specific societal conditions with the emergence of protest or its repression, it reveals less about the link between individuals and the specific movements in which they are involved, which is the core of this study.

Some social movement researchers focus on participation in social movements by comparing activists to nonactivists. The desired outcome of such comparisons is to isolate factors that differentiate activists from nonactivists. Consequently, the factors singled out are used to explain active participation in a social movement from nonparticipation.[25] These are not the questions I am trying to raise or answer.

My approach to AIDS and cancer activism is distinctively different from those frequently taken within social movement research. Instead of comparing women activists to women nonactivists or female to male activists, I focus exclusively on a comparison of women who are active in two different movements. My goal is to find underlying processes and lessons that we can learn from activists who are active within two movements that share differences and similarities.[26] My particular concern is the connection between activism and the various identities of these women. Finding how these connections work expands the existing explanatory framework within the social movement literature that explains recruitment and movement success in a broader context.

At the core of my inquiry are women activists who are involved in organizational responses to these two health care crises. How these women understand their activism and the meaning it has for them is presented in this book. To reach a deeper understanding of the activist women's identities and motivations, I utilize feminist theory and black feminist theory in particular. My approach to women's activism examines the specific resources that these women use for their involvement (chapter 3); how their motivations for involvement are connected to their self-identities (chapter 4); and which organizational cultural dynamics women created and how they are connected to collective identities (chapters 5 and 6).

I argue that examining these micropatterns provides valuable answers for the members of these two social movements. But they are also of interest for others who are outside of the AIDS and breast cancer movements. These microprocesses often hold movements together. They make movements inviting to certain constituencies but not necessarily to others. Thus, I maintain that an understanding of these subtle internal movement dynamics also determines a movement's ultimate success. Knowing that certain dynamics or a certain movement culture determines that a particular segment of the overall constituency is more likely to get involved than other segments is crucial for mobilizing and sustaining a movement. This knowledge regarding internal movement dynamics and the interaction between the constituency base and movement is an important contribution to the body of social movement literature. In addition, I argue that activists must be concerned about being cognizant of processes that can limit their success by undercutting their constituency base or by increasing their mobilization by expanding their constituency base.

Is it activism or volunteerism?

Women activists in the breast cancer or AIDS movements have social change goals connected to these two health crises. This focus clearly prioritizes the political aspects of involvement; this activism nevertheless can overlap with volunteerism. The understanding of the activist as an agent of political change differs from the common definition of the volunteer—an unpaid helper who provides services for others. Nevertheless, these terms are often used interchangeably. This is especially true in the context of the AIDS movement, in which volunteers often are the focus of studies.[27] The AIDS movement, as well as other movements, has demonstrated that providing services for members of one's community is a political act.[28] Therefore, I need to clarify that my focus is on activists instead of on volunteers.

We learn from Wendy Kaminer, who investigated women volunteerism, that volunteering has two meanings. "Political activism—organized protests against government policy and challenges to its authorities—are . . . a part of an American volunteer tradition. Volunteering is not just a charity but confrontation."[29] Immediately the AIDS movement comes to mind because it has given such ample evidence for both of these meanings. If this is so, then why not choose women who are volunteers as well as women who define themselves as activists? There are important reasons not to do so.

The meaning of volunteerism has changed over time. Depending on its meaning, it has a loaded connotation for certain groups. Two moments in recent history changed the meaning of volunteering and still affect today's perception of volunteers.

Under Ronald Reagan's presidency, volunteerism was exploited by the political Right to justify government cutbacks. The Right portrayed volunteerism as a charitable helping of others that was strongly encouraged. Simultaneously, the Right separated volunteerism from its progressive social change aspect.

In the 1970s, feminists attacked any service-oriented volunteering that did not entail a social change component. According to feminist analysis, such serving and helping of others was a practice that perpetuated sexism, since the women worked unpaid. In addition, feminists argued that it was also bad for the people "it purported to serve; social services would never be adequately funded as long as women provided them for free."[30]

Kaminer[31] points out that the feminist attack on service volunteering was launched by neither working-class nor minority women. Instead, white feminists from middle- and upper-class backgrounds who were historically the group that most likely volunteered their services were the ones who discredited volunteering as an occupation that is diminishing to women.[32]

These constructions of the meaning of volunteering point to two reasons that have led me to exclude volunteers from my sample. First, women who have a strong social change goal are less likely to portray themselves as volunteers, since volunteering has the connotation of being charitable. Second, limiting my focus to volunteers—women who work without pay—has the potential to exclude a lot of women—all of those who cannot afford to provide their services for free.[33] Thus I include women who work for salary under certain conditions (as I explain later) and exclude certain women who are volunteers. I exclude all volunteers defined as women who are motivated to help by taking on tasks such as shopping and cleaning for people with a disease—typical of an AIDS "buddy" or women who volunteer support services to women with cancer. This is not to say that this type of volunteerism is excluded because it provides direct services that are not political. To the contrary, I agree with lesbian cancer activist Jackie Winnow, who has explained the political content of cancer activism in the following words:

> Somebody who was putting together a *politics* of cancer anthology once asked me why she should include the Mautner Project because it was direct services to lesbians. I said, "If you don't understand why a direct service agency to lesbians is political, you don't really understand anything—you've just put together the anthology."[emphasis added][34]

However, we are almost 20 years into the AIDS epidemic with no end in sight, after this amount of time, large bureaucratic organizations have been created in response to AIDS, sometimes called the "AIDS service industry."[35] These organizations deal with advocacy as well. One respondent addressed the reasons for the change in organizational types:

> I feel like I am in a job and not just try to stave off the epidemic. Because it's almost somewhere along the line everyone has started to build these mammoth organizations because we know AIDS is gonna be around for a long time. There was a different feeling in the beginning, when you felt if you worked really hard maybe we could find a cure and maybe this wouldn't happen anymore, and I think that has really shifted. And I think that the AIDS movement has shifted with it and become more bureaucratized and more settled in like we gonna be here not just for a long haul but for the longest haul. Hm, maybe that's really affected some of how things have been shaped. [AIDS movement]

Even though breast cancer organizations are generally less bureaucratized, some organizational types have evolved that employ women to do advocacy work.[36]

My inquiry of women's goals and the cultural patterns that have been created within these two movements requires that I cover the entire spectrum from the unpaid to the employed activist. I argue that cultural patterns and goals within large bureaucratic organizations are more influenced by employed women who work full time on advocacy than by direct service volunteers. These full-time activists make decisions about boundaries for volunteers, act on behalf of the unpaid constituency, and are influential in the approach to and execution of certain tasks. This has led me to exclude all of those volunteers who are executing the tasks (direct services) that have been set up by others. I am opposed, however, to selecting only interviewees who are in leadership positions, because it would limit the breadth of activism to the dominant perspective.[37] Therefore, I have included leaders, organization members, women who have chosen AIDS or breast cancer as the arena for their political activism, and women who work for pay in the areas of AIDS or breast cancer.

How do we find activists?

I used three alternate strategies for finding women activists: The first involved locating women through organizations that I classified as activist organizations. Second, I approached women directly whom I perceived as activists while I attended various conferences, rallies, and so forth, as well as membership meetings of cancer and AIDS organizations. Third, I established a referral system by asking the women I interviewed for names of other activists I could interview.

When I approached women through organizations, I selected organizations that are gender mixed as well as women only. I considered activist organizations and organizations with an activist component. I excluded organizations such as AIDS hospices and cancer support groups whose goals are providing services and care to people with a disease. I did include women who worked within specific departments of AIDS service industry organizations, such as advocacy, education, policy, women's programs, and community programs, but I excluded the support programs such as buddy programs. I used the same selection process for cancer organizations: I included women who were involved in functions other than providing direct services.

I approached women directly when I perceived them as cancer or AIDS activists. These are women who have spoken on panels as representatives of a certain community or an organization or have served as consumer activists. The organizational approach indicated that I exclude service-oriented organizations. I did not, however, exclude women who were selected as activists due to their involvement in activist organizations or as spokespersons, even when I found out that these women also did additional volunteer work or direct services for a hospice or in organizations such as the American Cancer Society.

Who is an activist?

I interviewed thirty-seven women who had been selected according to these three methods.[38] Even though these methods were chosen to ensure that my respondents were activists, it did not ensure that the women defined themselves as activists. At times there was disagreement between my ascribing an activist label to women when the women themselves were not embracing this identity. Five respondents rejected the term *activist* for themselves. All five are women of color who are in paid positions, three in AIDS and two in breast cancer activism.[39] Activism has a political connotation for these women that they distinguish from their tasks or positions within AIDS or breast cancer.

> I consider myself a breast cancer provider. . . . [A]ctivist, that word sounds to me very political and I am not very involved in lobbying and [advocacy organization] and that sort of thing. I participate in [the advocacy organization's] activities but that is something personal. . . . I consider myself a voice for the Latino community. Because first of all there are not many people doing that kind of work, breast cancer work with Latinos or Latina women specifically. [cancer movement, woman of color]

Women of color see their work within the AIDS and breast cancer movements as different from an activism that centers around lobbying and protesting. One woman distanced herself from the term *activist* because her job put her on the inside of a system, whereas activism meant for her fighting for institutional change while she was outside of the system. The tasks these women perform are advocacy for women with disease, prevention, and education of their communities.

> I am committed to treatment, to high quality treatment for poor people. My background is in services of families of child abuse or battering. It's all about people who are in need. And typically services of poor people tend to be poor services. I am committed to believing that just because you are poor that does not mean that you should get poor services. That's where

> my commitment is. It's not to AIDS specifically. . . . My focus
> is primarily on poor people which in many cities is African
> American, but it's not always the case needless to say . . . social
> services is what I do. I don't know if that is activism, I don't
> have protest signs and all that stuff. I come in here everyday
> and I slog away the very, very unattractive work of trying to
> keep [things] afloat. [AIDS movement, woman of color]

These women see themselves primarily as professionals who are
working within a field in which poor people, women of color, or both,
are marginalized and mistreated by having no voice and little or no
access to services. All of these women serve as advocates for women
or marginalized communities.

These women point to an important problem with the connotation
of activism. Similar to the two existing definitions of volunteerism,
activism can also be understood in two ways. One meaning of activism is politics through protest and lobbying to accomplish institutional change. The second meaning is broader and defines activism as
a political change strategy through protest, lobbying, and so forth, but
it also includes advocacy on behalf of and providing services to the
disadvantaged.

While one definition of volunteerism portrays helping without
social change, one definition of activism suggests activism is protest
without care for the people. Kaminer, who interviewed volunteers,
writes:

> "What is a volunteer?" I asked . . . a thirty-two-year-old His-
> panic woman who works full time as the paid director of a
> community health center and as an unpaid "organizer." "Vol-
> unteers," she said, "are middle-aged white women coming in
> to help out. . . . They mean well, but they don't know what the
> hell they are doing."[40]

While focusing on activism, I have found the counterpoint to this
definition of volunteering. When I asked one woman of color, "What
is an activist?" she answered:

> For me the typical activist is one who lobbies, goes to the
> legislature, and protests, and walks and does all that stuff.
> And due to my schedule I have no time to do all of that.
> [cancer movement]

This woman did not go as far as to suggest that activists are white women who protest while she is busy providing services and advocating for her community. But it is not too far of a stretch to imagine that this partly underlies her definition of activism. Further, when I asked white women within the cancer movement, "Do you know of any cancer activists of color?", many answered, "Women of color are service providers but not activists." This indicates a connotation of activism as an enterprise by white people with resources.

I argue that a definition of activism has to be broad enough to cover the provision of needed services in combination with protest. In order to include women in different locations who perform different tasks in response to the AIDS and breast cancer crises, I use a definition of activism that combines advocacy, services, and political protest.

Is it breast cancer activism or cancer activism?

Activists have not always welcomed my focus on breast cancer activism, and there has been considerable debate at times about whether one should call it a "cancer" movement or a "breast cancer" movement. One group of activists favors putting the emphasis on "cancer" rather than "breast cancer." While everyone admits that breast cancer is the most prevalent form of cancer, one group of activists argues that women get all kinds of cancer. By calling it a breast cancer movement, this group argues, one separates women with breast cancer from women with other types of tumors. The second group of activists favors using "breast cancer" as the focal point without implying a separation or rejection of women with other types of cancer.

The debate is reflected within the names of the various cancer organizations. On the one hand, some organizations call themselves Women's Community Cancer Project (Cambridge, Massachusetts) or the Women's Cancer Resource Center (Berkeley, California). On the other hand, some organizations call themselves the Massachusetts Breast Cancer Coalition (Boston) or Breast Cancer Action (San Francisco).

This division is not easily explainable simply by saying that women who have breast cancer are the women who argue in favor of a "breast cancer" movement. To the contrary, many of the proponents of a women's "cancer" movement have breast cancer themselves. For instance, Susan Liroff, who has breast cancer, argues for "cancer" activism.

> In California, groups are forming to lobby for legislative relief and for more research money specifically for breast cancer. . . .

> We at the WCRC [Women's Cancer Resource Center] have
> some differences with these other groups because they limit
> the scope of attention to just breast cancer. It's certainly true
> that breast cancer is a major killer of women, but just recently
> we lost two women who were very close to our hearts to
> cervical cancer and Hodgkin's disease. . . . I think it would be
> a mistake for us to open the door to a financial or legislative
> "divide and conquer" routine—that is, the funding of research
> and/or resources for breast cancer only, excluding women who
> are stricken with other forms of the disease.[41]

Another woman with breast cancer, Jackie Winnow, also argues against
forming organizations that specifically target breast cancer.

> It's easier to organize around breast cancer . . . because no one
> can deny it's a women's and health issue and a lot of media
> alarm can be generated around it because women and their
> breasts are so tied together in this country. If you get into
> other cancers, you start to see more subtle ways women are
> controlled in this society and that gets more complicated.[42]

Counterarguments that favor a "breast cancer" movement vary in
their explanations. The "cancer" activists' accusations about separation are rejected, while the specificity of the relationship between breasts
and women's identity are highlighted. For instance, one activist I interviewed told me:

> [Having breast cancer] really affects who they are as women
> in their identity. . . . [At the] first rally we had, a woman came
> up to me, and she said, "You know, seven years ago, I had a
> mastectomy and six years ago, I had my other breast removed
> and I have never told anybody." She was always ashamed to
> tell anybody. She wouldn't have been ashamed if she had had
> part of her intestines removed or anything else. But her whole
> identity as a woman she did not know what to do with it.
> Women have had their husbands leave them because they had
> breast cancer or a mastectomy. It doesn't happen with other
> stuff. [cancer movement]

While this debate is ongoing, some of the self-identified "cancer"
organizations have joined umbrella organizations such as the National

Breast Cancer Coalition [emphasis mine]. Even though I started out with the intention of comparing "breast" cancer activism to AIDS activism, I decided to include women who understood themselves as "cancer" activists. Since cancer activists and breast cancer activists are not consistent and the division is not so deep to acknowledge two separate movements, I refer to the cancer and the breast cancer movement interchangeably.

Does health status make a difference?

Another issue under consideration is the respondents' health status. Cancer activists are depicted as women with the disease, but women AIDS activists are perceived as being political and HIV-negative (see chapter 3). Such a portrayal of activism frames cancer activism as self-interest, while AIDS activism is political. I argue against such a presentation of women's activism. I have included women who live with different diseases as well as activists who are without disease. In other words, I have included women who have breast cancer along with women who have another form of cancer. I also have included women without disease as well as women with HIV or AIDS. While women who live with breast cancer are not hard to find, this is not true for the AIDS movement. Studies that focus on male activists regularly include the opinions and perspectives of HIV-positive activists, but HIV-positive women are hardly ever represented as political subjects or activists. Therefore, I saw it as my task to include the voices of women with HIV or AIDS and to represent their perspectives on their activism.

Is sexual orientation important?

Last, but not least, I selected women activists according to their sexual orientation. My goal was to select an equal number of lesbian and straight women.[43] This automatically raised the question of how I defined a lesbian versus a straight woman. For the purpose of finding interviewees, I required only that women reveal their sexual identity. While sexual identity and sexual behavior are controversial issues addressed within this book, I went along with whatever identity a woman embraced for herself.

I argue that sexual orientation is an important issue that affects who we are and how we perceive ourselves in the world. When I asked women within the AIDS movement questions about sexual orientation, it was an accepted part of the conversation that did not appear to stand out from the other questions I raised. But within the breast cancer movement, questions about sexual orientation were not perceived so matter-of-factly. Many women, regardless of their own sexual identity, disagreed with me about the importance of discussing sexual orientation within the context of breast cancer.

There have been two lines of arguments that women put forward to reject the importance of sexual orientation within the breast cancer movement. One argument is similar to the debate that women have had about defining "cancer" and "breast cancer" activism. The women argue that we should not divide women by distinguishing lesbians from straight women. These women favor a movement that is inclusive of *all women*, regardless of their sexual orientation, type of cancer, or race or socioeconomic status. The counterargument states that breast cancer is not a sexually transmitted disease. Sexual behavior has no bearing on women's risk for cancer.

> [Sexual orientation is] not central. See, I think the difference is that one of the ways you can contract HIV is by behavior that is identified as being gay in terms of anal intercourse, etc., etc. So there is a more of a sexual orientation connection to gay men who work on the AIDS epidemic, I mean again, there is this, there is the issue of homophobia, there is the issue of denial of their chosen way to express their own sexuality. That's not the case with breast cancer. So the issue of sexual behavior is never questioned in terms of breast cancer. I think it would be different, for example, if some study came out and said that women who don't have heterosexual sex, women who don't have intercourse, have a higher rate of breast cancer, a higher incidence of breast cancer. I think then you would see more lesbians working in around the political issues of breast cancer. Because they would then be targeted because of their behavior. You know, all of you lesbians getting breast cancer, that's because you don't want to have sex with men. Which is what society is saying to gay men. [cancer movement]

I maintain, however, that sexual orientation is an important issue to address within the breast cancer and AIDS movements. Because many lesbians are activists in these movements, it is necessary to investigate how these women's sexual orientation affects and interacts with their activism in the two health crises. Since the social construction of AIDS has blurred the lines between sexual behavior and sexual identity, it is important to address this issue within activism. Further, evidence exists which suggests that lesbians have an increased risk of developing breast cancer compared to straight women, while their risk of contracting HIV is perceived as negligible. In this context, the lack of generalizable data on lesbian health and women's health studies' omission of questions about sexual orientation were criticized, therefore, this study of activism will consider sexual orientation.

What does this selection mean?

Having presented the vantage point from which I approach women's activism in the AIDS and breast cancer movements, as well as the selection criteria I used to include respondents, it poses the question of what the consequences of this vantage point and such a selection process are.

Selecting respondents according to my criteria has the following advantages. One is that I have focused on including voices that are usually less audible. By focusing on women without comparing them to men, women's concerns are at the center, and the multiplicity of women's lives becomes a more prominent feature.

Feminists have argued historically against the practice of using men as the default, making generalizations, and applying findings to women. While this opened the door to many studies that focused on gender by comparing female to male activists in various movements such as the civil rights and labor movements, it reinforces gender as a binary that constructs women's lives in comparison to men's. For this reason I have chosen not to compare women and men activists within the AIDS crisis or cancer's effects on women in comparison to men.

Other voices that are marginalized are HIV-positive women activists. These women are hard to find, and their voices are often omitted from the activism discourse. They are usually found within a discourse that focuses on controlling transmission and on the "victims" of AIDS. But this discourse renders women as objects, while I perceive women with HIV who are active about their disease as subjects.

Finally, using sexual orientation as another selection criterion gives credibility to the specificity of lesbians' lives. This perspective approaches sexual orientation as an issue that deserves more attention than it has usually been given within the AIDS and breast cancer movements, but also within the recent feminist literature. As Sarah

Schulman points out, "A new viciously homophobic feminism is emerging."[44] One example Schulman gives is Susan Falludi's much acclaimed book *Backlash*, which accomplishes the task to discuss women's oppression for 550 pages without mentioning the word "lesbian" once. This trend of not mentioning lesbians or rarely mentioning lesbians has been ongoing within important feminist health literature.[45] Frequently this occurs rather blatantly within books that discuss sexuality after mastectomy or breast reconstruction by focusing solely on husbands or male sexual partners.[46]

Other voices and the difference in experiences that have been examined are discrepancies in health and socioeconomic status and race. I argue that activism and the meaning it has for women are interlinked with identities, and so, depending on a woman's identity, activism can take on different forms.

A final word of caution

Due to the need of arguing certain points and maintaining a structure within this book, I have isolated certain aspects of this study and looked at them separately. By doing so, I have essentially arranged women's lives into specific identities as though it were possible to look at one element of a woman's life without considering all of the other elements simultaneously. Social science research is known for dividing lives into separate categories, producing an artificial separation of human experience. For the sake of research and to aid in focusing on certain arguments, we chop the complexity of human lives into smaller pieces so we can examine them under the microscope. I apologize for continuing in this tradition. Moreover, social scientists often separate women's lives into preexisting categories such as gender, class, race, and sexual orientation. Of course, these experiences cannot be separated. For example, it is impossible to walk down the street and determine exactly to which attributes we are reacting when a black, lesbian, HIV-positive mother from another country speaks out. Using the method of separation, which I am partially guilty of repeating, certain classic mistakes are committed and falsities are reinforced— such as lesbians are white, and everyone poor is of color. I hope that the reader can overlook the limitation of this approach and remember that our lives are much more complex and less orderly than I make them appear for the sake of making my theoretical points. I will occasionally remind the reader that we embody multiple identities that we do not experience separately.

CHAPTER 3

Two Worlds: The Political Culture of AIDS and Breast Cancer Activism

Being within an AIDS or a breast cancer setting is a different cultural experience. To capture the difference between these cultures, I have used the expression of the "two worlds." Even though I talk about "two worlds" or "different worlds," I also found a number of similarities between them. Within each movement there are certain processes that are similar. But these processes may take on a different form or importance within the AIDS or breast cancer culture. These processes and their differences and similarities are the main focus of this chapter.

Public perception of cancer and AIDS activists

The media's reporting on AIDS and breast cancer activism reflects the cultural differences between cancer and AIDS activists. Moreover, the media actively constructs the persona of "woman cancer activist," which is significantly different from the persona of the "woman AIDS activist." First I will present these constructed images and their differences, but underneath such apparent differences there is again a similarity: both groups of activists are inadequately presented in the media.

The Persona of the AIDS activist

The Women's Caucus of ACT UP sums up the available information about women in the AIDS crisis as follows: "[W]omen are most of the time completely invisible, face severe and sometimes insurmountable obstacles to coming out with a positive HIV status."[1] Contrary to invisibility, visibility is present merely for chosen public figures or icons. Such icons are important because they affect the public's perception of a social issue such as AIDS.

Rock Hudson's disclosure of having AIDS certainly marked a turning point in the history of the public's awareness of the disease. Furthermore, more dramatically for the African-American community, Magic Johnson's announcement that he was HIV-positive and Arthur Ashe's announcement that he had AIDS marked particular turning points. Women with HIV or AIDS are still deprived of an icon or a public image of a woman with HIV or AIDS who is also an activist. The only women who have attracted considerable media coverage due to their HIV status are Elizabeth Glaser (the wife of Hollywood filmmaker Paul Michael Glaser), and Mary Fisher (who spoke at the Republican National Convention in 1992). But these women are less known because they are less frequently reported on in the media and are also less well-known celebrities.[2] Therefore, these women's "going public" with their disease did not create a similar turning point in public awareness of women and AIDS as did the men's public announcement of their HIV/AIDS status. In addition, the class and race (upper class and white) of these female public figures are most likely also responsible for the extent to which the media reports on these women's serostatus. As Valerie Sacks points out:

> Despite the fact that rates of seropositivity among Western women are highest among lower-class black or Latina women, such women are also the least visible in discourses on AIDS. Rather, it is the middle-class white women—those who are statistically less likely to contract HIV and thus somewhat atypical AIDS victims—who appear most frequently.[3]

When the media does report on HIV-positive women, they are not depicted as activists. Quite to the contrary, women with HIV or AIDS are frequently portrayed as an adjunct to men. The portrayal of women reflects the double bind of being "victim" or "villain." On the one hand, women are seen as passive objects who get infected by men. On the other hand, they are threatening to men by infecting them and hence a danger for the "general population." Evelynn Hammonds argues that African-American women are omitted from the media's discourse on AIDS and also points out that, when African-American women are mentioned, their portrayal is biased.

> African-American women with AIDS are constantly represented with respect to drug use—either their own or their partners. They are largely poor or working-class. They are single mothers. Media portrayals of these people with AIDS allude to the specter of drug abuse and uncontrolled sexuality coupled with welfare "dependency" and irresponsibility. Such allusions undermine any representations of African-American women with AIDS that would allow them to be embraced by the larger public.[4]

Hence, women with AIDS or HIV-positive women are generally excluded from a public discourse in that they are not consulted for AIDS reporting and are not perceived as acting subjects or activists.[5] This creates a situation that women with AIDS or HIV-positive women are less visible than men and virtually nonexistent as AIDS activists, while they are portrayed as "AIDS victims" or "villains" who contribute to the spread of the disease. Chris Norwood, who has studied the print media's coverage of AIDS with regard to women, concludes:

> In general, media coverage of women and AIDS has been so replete with sexist, racist and class assumptions, but so bereft of basic, factual information, that the press itself has come to play a defining role in the women's part of the epidemic which can only be described as unethical.[6]

Nevertheless, the media has created a persona of a woman "AIDS activist." The media's construction of a "woman AIDS activist or a spokesperson" is a woman who is not infected with the virus. Some famous women come to mind, such as Elizabeth Taylor, who became active early on raising money for AIDS services for people with the disease. A second group of uninfected women who are active with AIDS issues is the activist who is assumed to be a lesbian. Both types of AIDS activists share the creation of an impression that these women are active on behalf of men with AIDS. Notably missing in the public discourse are women AIDS activists, regardless of serostatus, who are

committed to their cause of benefiting women with AIDS and of preventing uninfected women from contracting HIV.

The Persona of "cancer activist"

In comparison, what is the media's portrayal of women who have
breast cancer? Cancer has existed longer as a disease, and throughout
the disease's history a number of public figures have drawn attention
to their breast cancer diagnoses.[7] My focus, however, is on the media's
construction of the "cancer activist," not on women with cancer.

The media created the persona activist as a woman who is active
due to her cancer diagnosis. Cancer activists are never presented as
being active for reasons other than perceived self-interest due to their
cancer. In terms of cancer activists' political background, commonly
the following explanatory framework is put forward. On the one hand,
women with cancer are portrayed as first-time activists. On the other
hand, women's cancer activism is explained as an outcome of the
aging "baby boomer" generation, since women of this age group are
more prone to developing cancer. Since the baby boomer generation is
associated with the political activism of the 1960s and 1970s, it is argued that they have decided to face the disease with the means they
learned during their politically active years during these decades. To
show that women's cancer activism is publicly framed as evolving
from the hands of first-time activists and also based on the political
activism of the 1960s as well, I refer to an article in the *New York Times*
in 1993. The article marks a turning point in the public's awareness of
breast cancer activism due to the picture of a woman with a mastectomy that appeared on the cover of *New York Times Magazine*.[8] Susan
Ferraro, the author of the article, drew upon both explanatory frameworks. First she begins her article by creating the type of a woman
who is new to political activism but driven to it in anger. Along with
the breast cancer diagnosis, the attitudes of the medical establishment
with which she came into contact while undergoing her treatment
made her angry. She consequently turned to activism.

> "I was never political, never," says LoRusso, a home econom-
> ics teacher who is on disability leave. She lives in Huntington,
> LI, in a pleasant two-story ranch, and chauffeurs her two kids
> after school, runs errands and frets about dinner and dust. "I
> was the peacemaker, the people pleaser. I had 16 years of
> Catholic school. The nuns said 'Jump.' I said, 'How high?' "

Liz LoRusso is less obedient now. She has joined 1 in 9, an advocacy group that takes its name from a commonly quoted statistic on the incidence of breast cancer.[9]

A few pages later, Ferraro presents a second type of cancer activist by linking cancer activism to the political background of a certain age group.

Certainly, one thing the movement has going for it is timing— noisy 1960's activists who are in their 40's and 50's and baby boomers who were nursed on 60's activism are increasingly at risk for breast cancer. They understand the power of group politics. "I wasn't a *famous* [emphasis in original] activist, but I protested the war in the 60's," says Visco, the breast cancer coalition's president. "I spoke out for women's rights in the '70's."[10]

Even though the political background of the "cancer activist" is diverse in that first-time activists and 1960s' activists are both depicted as being part of the movement, class and race are less diverse. The media's depiction of a "woman cancer activist" is white and middle- or upper-class. Missing is the image of cancer activists who do not have the disease themselves. As is the case for AIDS as well, there are also omitted public images of women who come from backgrounds other than white and middle-or upper-class.

This presentation of the media's portrayal of breast cancer and AIDS activists prepares the ground for a more in-depth discussion of two issues. First it has touched on important themes such as gender, race, class, sexual orientation, and health status, which are played out differently within an AIDS or a cancer environment. But, second, it shows a similarity: there are missing images within the media's portrayal of both AIDS and breast cancer activists.

SECTION 3.1 NEW ACTIVISTS

There are first-time activists in both the cancer and the AIDS movements. Not having prior activist experience should be a commonality that makes these women alike, even though they represent different movements. Furthermore, the political newcomers in cancer and AIDS activism are both living with a disease.[11]

Timing of activism when living with a disease

Superficially, women who are HIV-positive and women who have cancer seem to share the commonality of living with a life-threatening illness, and they become active regarding their disease after they have been diagnosed. But there are various differences between the diseases themselves that affect the opportunity or the timing of women's involvement in activism. The progression of each disease determines the window of opportunity for involvement differently. That is, frequently women who tested positive for HIV get involved after they have been tested and not when they are sick. So HIV-positive women's involvement tends to be at a time when they may feel physically strong and perceive themselves as fit and healthy because they do not suffer from an AIDS-related illness. Women who are diagnosed with cancer, however, often have no opportunity to get involved in cancer organizing right after their diagnosis because the disease takes a different course. In many cases, a cancer diagnosis means surgery, followed by a variety of treatment choices that require different time commitments. Since six months of chemotherapy treatment after a breast cancer diagnosis and surgery is common, a woman with that course of medical treatment will often not have the opportunity to get involved until she has completed chemotherapy, which can be almost one year after her initial diagnosis.[12] Therefore, the progression and treatment of the disease create different conditions for the timing of women's involvement. A woman who is HIV-positive generally gets involved while she is living with the threat of a future defined by HIV-related infectious diseases.[13] In contrast, for the woman with cancer, involvement becomes more possible when the immediate physical aspects of the disease and its treatment are over, that is, at a time when many women feel that they are done with cancer.

Becoming active for the first-time

Women with HIV/AIDS have generally had no "political experience." Because they are new to advocacy and political activism, one assumes that their case is similar to that of first-time cancer activists. Contrary to what might be expected of these two groups, both of them new to activism and living with a disease, they actually turn out to be different with regard to socioeconomic and racial background. This is not to say that financially secure women are spared from HIV/AIDS, or that poor women do not develop breast cancer.[14] I have not found women among the cancer activists, however, who come from poor backgrounds and who have turned their cancer diagnosis into activism. Within cancer activism, I have found women of color, but they are not poor and have no cancer diagnosis. Within AIDS, however, being poor and of color is frequently the background of HIV-positive women; they turned to activism after their positive HIV test result. Thus one specific culture within the AIDS environment, a "poor culture," exists, which is different from and coexists with the culture many gay men created. I will discuss these cultural aspects in more detail later within the context of collective identity. Despite the racial and economic differences between cancer and AIDS activists, there is also one similarity: AIDS and cancer activism have attracted and politicized new groups of women, women who have never before been active.

Skills of first-time activists

The existence of economic and social differences between seropositive first-time AIDS activists and first-time cancer activists has different implications. Even though both groups have no prior experience in activism, the HIV/AIDS activists' accounts are filled with references to a prior history of fighting for their survival. This is exemplified through the words of one HIV-positive AIDS activist, who recalls that every step in her life required her to fight.

> So I think what I started realizing once I got into recovery [from substance abuse] that everything was a fight for women. I had to fight to get my son back. Once I got my son back, I had to fight for housing. At the time, I couldn't go into a shelter because my son had [an illness]. . . . I am thinking, here I am in recovery, I wasn't even clean a year, had to get my son back, couldn't afford housing. I had a job as a receptionist. I had dropped out of school. I had no degrees. I had nothing. And I had to keep fighting. . . . I got a section 8, I got my son back. I had to fight for daycare, I had to fight for everything. And that's when I started noticing that all women have to fight. But what it showed me was that me learning how to use the tools, gave me tools to use for other women. So I think that was my calling on becoming an activist. So that was the beginning of it. [AIDS movement, woman of color, HIV-positive]

AIDS activism is framed here as merely a slight variation on what she had done all along—fight for her survival.

Due to the socioeconomic background of women with HIV/AIDS, coming to political awareness is not perceived as "a moment of enlightenment,"[15] in that the seropositivity and the activism that ensued caused them to experience the world as unjust in terms of power imbalances. I interviewed many women who indicated that finding out that they are HIV-positive was more of the same, just one more struggle for survival. Many published accounts also express this point as well.

Who has survival skills?

It is impossible to distinguish this argument further by race, class, and sexual orientation. All of the HIV-positive women I interviewed were poor and some were lesbians, but I interviewed only one white woman with HIV/AIDS. I therefore argue that these survival skills within the context of AIDS are rooted in a *marginal* culture. They stem from belonging to a counterculture or subculture that has forced its members to develop skills of survival and resistance from a seemingly powerless social position. The women activists who are HIV-positive come from communities that are marginal. The women have come to use their survival skills within an AIDS context. Outside of AIDS, survival skills have been acknowledged to exist among other marginal communities, such as women of color, lesbians, prostitutes, and substance abusers.[16]

Within the AIDS environment, the survival skills that first-time activists bring to their activism can function as a possible connection to other women AIDS activists. Even though other AIDS activists are different with regard to their health status, their political experience and class background connect them to the HIV-positive activists who come from disenfranchised backgrounds. One avenue of connection is that some of the seronegative activists stem from subcultures in which those survival skills are rooted; they are lesbians, women of color, or both. Another link that I will discuss later is the fact that politically experienced AIDS activists have mostly gained their political experience from movements that focus on gender, class, race, and sexual orientation—the issues that determine the first-time activists' disenfranchisement and their lifelong struggle against it.

Further, that women with HIV/AIDS turn their survival skills into first-time activism is directly related to the longevity of AIDS activism and AIDS organizations. Many AIDS organizations have developed programs that seek to empower women with HIV/AIDS.[17] At this point, similar empowerment programs are nonexistent among the cancer movement, which means that women with cancer have to make their first step into an unfamiliar political arena by using their own devices.

Programs that ease the way of women into cancer activism are emerging within the cancer movement as well. On a national level, the National Breast Cancer Coalition (NBCC) offers two programs. One is an advocacy training program that teaches women how to lobby, among other things. The second program is called Project Lead, which is taught by scientists and clinicians to prepare women to be informed consumer activists who can understand and comprehend scientific cancer research studies. The program is designed to enable women to become involved on research boards that decide which research applications will get funding. But both programs clearly cater to women who have a certain educational level[18] and moreover to women who have the economic resources that allow them to participate.[19]

Differences in skills

First-time cancer activists also have skills or tools at their disposal, but these skills are very different in comparison to the tools and the survival skills of first-time AIDS activists. Nevertheless, first-time activists in both AIDS and breast cancer mobilize personal resources when confronted with the life-threatening illness that has brought them into activism.

I define "personal resources"[20] as the crucial tools or skills that make us who we are in the world or that we use in order to relate to or make sense of the world around us. Hence, the women who enter into activism call on their personal resources because they enter into and experience a new environment of which they need to make sense. These skills cover a wide variety of things and range on a continuum from behavior to material resources. Our social position determines the range of personal resources that are available to us. Our social location depends on race, class, gender, sexual orientation, nationality, and ethnic origin.[21]

I have already introduced the concept of survival skills for HIV-positive women activists. Exactly what these skills are can be exemplified with the account of one HIV-positive woman. This ex-offender uses the technique she once used for selling drugs and now uses it for AIDS and safer-sex peer education. She is aware that the strengths and skills she attributes to her background as a substance abuser stem from her parents, who were substance abusers. She uses these skills today as an activist to the benefit of her former peers, substance-abusing women.

> It's like selling something. . . . I was selling for so many years but negative. I sold drugs. That's why I was incarcerated, because I sold drugs for so many years. So the same technique, and that same style, I use it positive now. You see, I don't really have to start new, a new life. I just have to modify and smooth in the rough edges of the ones that I already have. . . . [M]y past made me who I am today. Maybe good or bad, it's who I am today. My distorted family, my abusive background of my father's drug use. Whatever it is, it made me the caring, understanding, rough, nasty, manipulative, reserved, little girl that I am today. [She talks about drug users who are shut down and refuse to listen when she tries to talk to them about the HIV virus.] [I]t's on me now, the little criminal that I am, I come and pick your locks. Get the glass cutter, cut the glass in the windows and open them all up, get in and do something positive and turn on the lights, go and find somebody home. So that's how I look at it. It's a good strategy, but it's messed up because I have to be the criminal for this to happen. But I can use that potential. [AIDS movement, HIV-positive]

There is a vast discrepancy in resources between first-time AIDS activists and first-time cancer activists, grounded in the different social strata from which women cancer activists come. Cancer activists have more socioeconomic resources at their disposal and, generally speaking, the cancer movement's culture is anything but "marginal." Whereas women activists with HIV/AIDS come from disenfranchised backgrounds, first-time women cancer activists use other resources that are available to them, which are often resources that stem from privilege.

The personal resources that first-time cancer activists use depend on the individual woman's social position. Hence the first-time cancer activists use resources that are available to white middle-class women. Such resources are education, income, a sense of empowerment or entitlement, and access to influential institutions or people in powerful positions within the legislature, politics, or health institutions. Despite these obvious differences in terms of the background of cancer activists and AIDS activists, the two groups share an underlying similarity. Both groups of women had no prior political experience and moved into activism because AIDS or cancer radicalized them.

Interaction between skills and external conditions

The use of resources is also assisted by certain external conditions. I have touched earlier upon this point within the AIDS movement by discussing empowerment programs that coach women from impoverished backgrounds on becoming activists. Resources such as access to influential institutions that cancer activists use have been assisted by certain external conditions as well.

First-time and experienced activists for breast cancer, were confronted with other conditions than AIDS activists who had started their struggle 10 years earlier. AIDS activists have been fighting vigorously for many years, and one of their successes has been to create change within the health arena. I am referring here to changes such as the conducting of and access to drug trials, the speed with which drugs are approved, and the creation of a dialogue between activists and pharmaceutical industries, as well as a willingness by major health institutions such as the CDC to meet with health activists. In the early 1990s, when breast cancer activists obtained media attention and cancer grassroots groups were mushrooming all over the country, the response to breast cancer activism was different due to the window of opportunity that had been created by AIDS activism.

The breast cancer activists were "courted" to a certain degree by the establishment. One activist recalls,

> It was a fascinating experience to be involved with power and to be close to power. I did a lot of the Washington stuff and I went to NIH. It was the most exciting thing to go to the NCI and meet these people, to see this whole world of research and then we got toured around. They wanted us to like them better than the AIDS people had liked them. So they really tried with the cancer activists. We had a big meeting our leadership and the NCI, the whole staff of NCI met with the activists. [cancer movement]

Thus, in addition to having more resources available than AIDS activists, cancer activists were faced with a different societal condition, created to a certain degree from the doors that the AIDS activists had opened. It is a multilayered interaction: on the one side, there are doors that were opened for cancer activists, and on the other side, cancer activists also came with the appropriate tools and resources for the dialogue that took place behind these doors. These tools and skills are white middle-class ones necessary for being invited into dialogues with government institutions and health power brokers.

Meaning of first-time activism in women's lives

Becoming politically involved within cancer activism has a different position in women's lives than AIDS activism. First-time AIDS activists see their activism as just one more struggle in addition to the many other struggles and injustices they have experienced in their lives. To demonstrate the difference in women's perceptions of their lives, I like to quote one first-time woman cancer activist who reviews her life as follows:

> [Being diagnosed with breast cancer] was obviously one of the most significant events in my life, but it was also one of the most positive or awakening events in my life to realize that I wasn't doing anything in my life prior to this. I was just going along working and not getting really into any issues, always sort of staying on the outside of issues or political arenas. I realized after all of this that you can't do that. You've got to participate in life, in issues. To do what I was doing before, I was just existing. This is how significant a change it has been in my life: I went from a wallflower to being very prominent in the middle of a room. I no longer feel that my opinion doesn't matter because it really does matter. I feel I can say things now that I'd never thought about and actually have somebody give a response to it. I didn't feel entitled to that before. [cancer movement]

This cancer activist's account stresses the significance of the change that has taken place in her life. Making demands, being treated unfairly, and struggling politically is completely new, an awakening, and contradictory to what she experienced before in her life. This is not to claim that all first-time activists within the cancer movement are well off and that all was well in these women's lives prior to their cancer diagnoses. On the contrary, this cancer activist points to the fact that she lacked entitlement and a voice prior to her activism. Nevertheless, a difference remains between first-time cancer and AIDS activists.

Cancer activists' social position is more privileged in comparison to AIDS activists' and seems to have gone along with a lack of political framework or analysis for larger issues of injustice within society such as gender, race, class, and sexual orientation.

Another difference between first-time AIDS and cancer activists is that first-time AIDS activists were found only among HIV-positive women, whereas first-time cancer activists were found among women both with and without the disease.

Gay men and cancer activists

One can generalize that the gay men who started AIDS activism in the early 1980s share their race and socioeconomic makeup with the women cancer activists of the 1990s. Lack of political involvement, social location, and racial makeup characterize first-time cancer activists and clearly distinguish these women from first-time women AIDS activists. But these characteristics are similar to an earlier generation of first-time AIDS activists—gay men.

Within several historical accounts of the emergence of the AIDS movements, repeated references are made about the background of many gay men who became involved within AIDS activism. Within the beginning of the AIDS movement, two components came together. On the one hand, it has been widely documented that the response to AIDS has been spearheaded by the gay and lesbian community by using their existing organizational resources to build AIDS organizations. On the other hand, it is documented that many of the gay men who joined and formed early AIDS organizations were white, had no prior political interest or awareness, but became radicalized by the disease. Randy Shilts and Dennis Altman both describe that many gay men—for instance, those who founded the first AIDS organization, the Gay Men's Health Crisis (GMHC) in New York City— had never been active in gay politics before. They were deeply immersed in the "gay lifestyle" but had never been part of gay politics.[22] Gay men who had shied away from the politics of gay and lesbian liberation joined the AIDS movement as their first political involvement. This continued to happen later, as in the case of Michelangelo Signorile, who described himself as having come from the "gay party circuit" to ACT UP.[23]

To that extent, first-time activists, whether gay men or women within breast cancer activism, share similarities. Both groups have been radicalized by an epidemic that affects either themselves or someone close to them—a friend, lover, or family member. Second, these two groups share a similar race and socioeconomic makeup.

The portrayal of first-time activists within breast cancer activism differs from first-time cancer activists due to these women's socioeconomic background. Others might challenge the described class difference and suggest instead that the observed difference is due to a biased sample in which breast cancer activists with working-class backgrounds have been underrepresented. On the one hand, one response to this is that neither the AIDS nor breast cancer activists are representative of both movements in a statistical sense. On the other hand, I also argue that the observed class difference appears to be consistent with the groups of women who are most affected by either AIDS or breast cancer. Like any infectious disease, AIDS affects predominantly the disadvantaged within society. Therefore, it has to be understood as a disease that intersects race, class, gender, and sexual orientation. I am not aware of definite generalizable data on the socioeconomic status of women both with breast cancer and HIV disease, however, institutions such as the National Cancer Institute report that women of higher socioeconomic status tend to have higher rates of breast cancer,[24] and the CDC mentions that minority women are overrepresented among HIV-infected women and that these women tend to be poor.[25]

More important is the fact that my arguments are not rooted in numbers. Actually it might be that there is a sizable portion of women within cancer activism who do not have middle-class backgrounds. But since class is not discussed and the goals and assumptions of middle-class women are not challenged, the general impression is that it is a middle-class movement. Hence, I am arguing that the culture of the cancer movement is dominated by middle-class values, whereas the AIDS movement is more inclusive of a marginal culture. In chapters 5 and 6, I discuss in more detail how these similarities take shape within the movement environment and inform the style with which women cancer activists and AIDS activists pursue their goals.

SECTION 3.2 ACTIVISTS WITH POLITICAL EXPERIENCE

Racial, socioeconomic differences and the resources that are available to different groups have been discussed in order to present AIDS as a marginal culture and cancer as a white middle-class culture. Next, the political background and culture of these two movements is presented. Besides first-time activists who have become radicalized by an epidemic, there are of course in both movements activists who have gravitated toward AIDS or cancer but who have had prior political experience in other social movements.

Discussing and acknowledging these activists' political background are important for two reasons. First, these women's political experiences inform and guide their present activism. These women bring with them another set of skills than first-time activists. They bring their political savvy, knowledge, and loyalty to a set of political issues. Second, women's political background or loyalty to political issues creates a culture within the movements in much the same way the skills of the first-time activists create a certain culture.

Overall, women activists within the AIDS movement are different from activists in the cancer movement. As indicated earlier, one difference is the activists' health status. Politically experienced women in the AIDS movement are seronegative, whereas politically experienced cancer activists can be found among women with and without the disease. But more important, the activists also have different political agendas or histories, depending upon whether they are part of AIDS or cancer activism.

Generally, the HIV-negative women AIDS activists can look back on prior progressive involvement that informs their present political views while they are active within the AIDS movement. The only significant difference among AIDS activists is in regard to women's age. Younger AIDS activists have progressive politics, but, due to their age, they have less actual movement experience when compared to women AIDS activists in their forties, who describe their political activism in terms of a "solid, left-wing career." A woman in her forties recounts her political history as follows:

> I have a long history [of activism]. The first kind of political movement that I was involved in was the civil rights movement in the late '60s. I dropped out of college and got involved as an activist in civil rights work and then anti-war work, and then the beginning of the women's movement, and then through coming out in the gay and lesbian liberation. So I sort of had a pretty standard left-wing career of being involved in different movements and organizations that were sort of supporting this. I was a union activist for a long time, I was active as a union organizer. I was always involved in women's health care stuff. [AIDS movement, HIV-negative, in her forties]

Younger activists within the AIDS movement have the same emphasis on political issues such as gender, race, class, and sexual orientation, but they have spent less time being involved in movements such as the labor union or student movement. This age distinction applies to women AIDS activists of color as well.

Women of color articulate their political experience differently, however. They locate themselves first and foremost within their communities or, depending upon their age, within the context of the civil rights movement. A self-ascribed political location to the left of the political continuum is commonly not what women of color choose to express their political background. This is true even if they have been involved in the same movements (civil rights movement, anti-war movement, women's movement, gay and lesbian movement) as the white women, who end up calling themselves progressives. Women of color experienced racism within these progressive movements. Having encountered racism while being active in these movements makes them less of an ideological home for women of color, whereas they have successfully become a home for white women. Women of color locate themselves within their communities and tend not to take on the self-perception of progressives that white women have embraced.

Politically experienced cancer activists

The differences between politically experienced AIDS activists and cancer activists are prominent. AIDS activists' political culture can be summarized as a combination of first-time activists among the HIV-positive women, plus politically experienced women of color and progressive white activists. Cancer activists' political background is not as easy to categorize. Cancer activists vary with regard to their previous political involvements, as well as their political convictions. Cancer activists' political culture includes everything from first-time cancer activists to progressive seasoned activists similar to those found within AIDS politics. Cancer activists' political convictions span from liberals to conservatives. Due to the broadness of political range among cancer activists' political convictions, it is tempting somehow to distinguish the political culture of cancer activists.

It has been argued that women without cancer are more political and have more of an analysis than women with cancer. Supposedly, women without the disease are politically savvy and are active because of their political beliefs. In contrast, newcomers to activism are believed to be only among activists with cancer. I argue against this assumption, since I have encountered political newcomers with and without cancer. One cancer activist who had been involved in the cancer movement from the beginning characterized her political beliefs by pinpointing the dominant political conviction as a form of liberalism:

> I think that there are a lot of liberals in the cancer movement. . . . In fact, probably most, probably 95% of the women in the cancer movement, would describe themselves as liberals. So I am making a distinction between the left and liberals. I mean I remember that someone told me that somebody in the National Breast Cancer Coalition was a Republican. [cancer movement]

Whereas this characterizes the political conviction that is dominant within cancer, the actual political background of women who hold these beliefs is less easy to pinpoint. The range includes the activism of feminism and women's health, communities of color, the anti-war movement, gay and lesbian liberation, the environment, and activists for a responsible science. This raises the question of how it is possible that women, some of whom have a similar background to women within AIDS activism, can be part of a movement whose political culture can be characterized as liberal, even though some women have a progressive political background.

I suggest that this is an outcome of a number of things. I assume that the numeric distribution between women with progressive politics and experience on the one hand and women without political expertise on the other hand is skewed to the disadvantage of the politically progressive.[26] This assumption is informed by the fact that the women who have had prior progressive involvement indicated that within the movement there is little to no discussion around issues such as requirements for leadership. In fact, a woman with no prior political experience can achieve powerful or prominent leadership positions within the cancer movement.

Building connections

As indicated earlier, a process within the AIDS environment is the bridging or connecting between the group of disenfranchised activists and the progressive activists. Such bridging or connecting is possible because the HIV-negative progressive activists either stem from the

same subculture as the HIV-positive disenfranchised first-time activists (e.g., lesbians, communities of color) or have been involved within
movements that worked toward an end of oppression of these subcultures (e.g., civil rights movement). This indicates that connections or
bridging differences between groups of activists are made possible by
uniting around the theme of oppression.

It is therefore no surprise that a connection within cancer activism
takes on a completely different form. The connection among cancer
activists is based on sharing gender oppression. Most women cancer
activists, with or without prior political background, appear to come
from the dominant race and class makeup, which is white and middle
class. A recent publication confirmed the dominance of white and
middle class women by stating that among the 300 or so breast cancer
activist organizations are approximately 2 grassroots breast cancer activist groups organized by and for women of color.[27] The cancer activists, therefore, unite exclusively around their shared gender. However,
connecting based on the gender oppression that white middle-class
women share is a different climate than the bridging and unity among
AIDS activists who draw on their oppression due to race and class as
well as sexual orientation.

Conclusion

The two worlds of AIDS and cancer are different to the extent that
AIDS activism works with and caters to impoverished groups, whereas
the cancer movement's culture thrives on white middle-class values,
tools, and resources. The implications of such differences in movement culture are further discussed in chapters 5 and 6, which focus on
identity, diversity, and movement strategies.

Within the two worlds, some processes within each movement
have been shown to be similar. There is the new constituency that
both movements have among their activists—the first-time activists.
Another similarity is the process with which these first-time activists
make sense of their activism by using the resources or skills available
to them. Further, the culture within each movement is created by an
interaction among a diverse group of activists who unite around the
theme of oppression and bridge or overcome their existing differences.

CHAPTER 4

The Personal and the Political

Becoming involved in the AIDS or breast cancer movement is explainable by preconceived notions of women's motivations. In chapter 3, I discussed the public images of the breast cancer activist and the AIDS activist. Integrated within this constructed image of an "activist persona" are the perceived motivations for women to become active. One of these notions is self-interest.[1] Women who live with cancer are perceived as being motivated by their own self-interest. Within the AIDS movement, the common perception is that gay men become active due to their self-interest, whereas women AIDS activists are perceived as being active on behalf of men. Contrary to these two perceptions—self-interest on the one hand, and solidarity with men on the other hand—I argue that women's motivations are a combination of a personal and a political relationship to the disease. Further, I argue that the existence of just one of the two connections, either personal or political, is not sufficient to motivate women to activism.

In the case of women in the AIDS movement, solidarity[2] can be a motivating force; however, it is wrong to narrow it to solidarity with men. Further explaining activism as an outcome of solidarity is not specific enough. We are constantly surrounded by social problems and are often confronted with people in crises. Some of these move us enough that we take the step of becoming active on behalf of others, whereas other crises do not generate such a motivating force. Hence using solidarity as an explanation for activism omits the reasons why we are in solidarity with one group instead of another. Therefore, I argue that whenever activism is explained as being rooted in solidarity, we also need to explain the relationship of these groups of people to us and on whose behalf we are active.

There are many ways to respond to the argument of self-interest. One is to take the argument, embrace it, and hope that self-interest has a powerful impact.[3] But if this were the case, there would be more people involved in both movements, because the number of women who have lived or who are living with cancer or AIDS greatly exceeds the number of women who have been or who are active. This reference to numbers makes it clear that self-interest cannot be the only predictor for involvement; instead, it raises the question about what the motivations are for involvement.

Because of these reasons, self-interest and solidarity are not satisfying explanations of activism in either the AIDS or the breast cancer movement. My explanation for women's mobilization is instead that when women have a personal and a political relationship to the disease they become active. The personal and political relationship to the disease can be broken down into the following three motivational approaches: (1) diagnosis; (2) community activism; and (3) political-ideological approach to AIDS or breast cancer.

These three approaches can be thought of as ideal motivational types, three different interpretative frameworks that explain women's motivations to activism. I generated these motivational types inductively from the variety of reasons my respondents mentioned as their motivations for activism. Each motivational type combines women's political and personal relationships to the disease. The combination of the personal and the political varies, however, between types with regard to the intensity or dominance of the personal and the political.

The three motivational types have been created to understand the differences in motivations. Some women activists might apply more than one ideal type to themselves. In that sense, the ideal types of motivational forces are not mutually exclusive. The ordering of women into one motivational type versus another depends not on "objective facts," such as being diagnosed with a disease, being a certain race, having a certain sexual orientation, or having political experience. Instead, the ordering depends entirely upon women's subjective narratives and how they reasoned about their having become activists. For instance, a woman living with a disease might explain that this was not her motivating factor to become active around the disease, so she might argue that her motivation to activism was an outcome of her community activism or a logical step due to her political-ideological convictions.

The first ideal type, diagnosis, applies to women who start off with a personal relationship to the disease and then develop a political relationship as well, and the combination of the two brings these women to activism. At the core of this ideal type is the change of women's personal identity from being healthy to having a new self-identity of living with the disease. Triggered by a change in their health status, women undergo the transition from one personal identity to a new personal identity. These women's identity transformation is due to a changed health status, but the women also adopt to a more political identity, one that embraces a collective identity. This means that a woman's personal identity moves simply from being a woman with a disease to a collective identity of being an activist around a disease.

The second ideal type, community activism, applies to women whose personal identities are already overlapping with collective identities. This type applies, for instance, to a lesbian who identifies as a lesbian (personal identity) but who also embraces the collective identity of the gay and lesbian community (anti-homophobia). This is different from the identity of activists of the previous ideal type. Covered by the first ideal type are, for instance, the gay men, whom I discussed in chapter 3.[4] Even though these men had the personal identity of being gay, they became radicalized by a disease that affected their community, and they consequently developed a collective identity (anti-homophobia).

The third ideal type applies to activists who have been motivated predominantly by a collective identity. These activists' personal identities do not necessarily have to match their collective identities, for example, white women (personal identity) who embrace anti-racism (collective identity). This category could also be applied to straight women (personal identity) who embrace anti-homophobia (collective identity of the gay and lesbian community).

For clarity, I portray the ideal types as three separate entities. Some of the interviewed activists share, in reality, more of the elements that constitute specific ideal types. For instance, a lesbian who lives with cancer and has a strong environmental agenda is hard to confine to one motivational ideal type. There was no specific formula that I used to dissect this woman's responses regarding her motivations and with which I determined whether she belonged to ideal type one, two, or three. This woman's multiple-motivated activism was certainly not a good starting place in trying to make sense of women's motivations to activism, hence the ideal types emerged from those activists' narratives that entailed a clear, definable, singular motivation. As soon as the three ideal types were in place, they could explain all women's accounts of motivations to activism, even though some women's accounts do not neatly fit into a single ideal type.

In the presentation of the three ideal types, I focus on the differences between them and their commonality—the two components, a personal and a political relationship to the disease. In the discussion of the ideal types, I touch on collective identity, but I focus on this in more detail in chapters 5 and 6.

Section 4.1 Diagnosis

Women who are mobilized by a diagnosis are often first-time activists. Of course, this is not to say that a politically experienced woman cannot be diagnosed with a disease. To the contrary, politically experienced women have been diagnosed with breast cancer and have launched the breast cancer movement. My goal, however, is to distinguish among women's motivations for activism and not among women's health statuses, hence I differentiate between women's rationale for becoming active. Whereas one group claims that they have been motivated to activism by their politics (see Section 4.3), another group claims that they have been motivated by their diagnoses.

Being diagnosed

Anthony Giddens' notion of self-identity is helpful in understanding the effects of a diagnosis on the self:

> "The body" sounds a simple notion, particularly as compared to concepts like "self" or "self-identity." The body is an object in which we are all privileged, or doomed, to dwell, the source of feelings of well-being and pleasure, but also the site of illnesses and strains. However, as has been emphasized, the body is not just a physical entity which we "possess," it is an action-system, a mode of praxis, and its practical immersion

in the interactions of day-to-day life is an essential part of the sustaining of a coherent sense of self-identity.[5]

Therefore, having cancer or testing positive for HIV is more than a medical event, it also gives someone a new identity. The disease-stricken (or infected) person turns into one of "them"—a member of the group of the "unwell." A cancer diagnosis or a positive HIV test result is a life-changing event. As is typical for life-changing events, women remember the date when the event took place, some even the time of day and other inconsequential details. Women who have experienced this change delineate their lives into the time before and the time after the event took place. These women's new identity and the personal experience of living with a disease is something they turn into political activism with the motivation to spare others from also experiencing the disease. Within this group of women who turn to activism after they have been diagnosed, I distinguish between regular diagnosis and misdiagnosis.

Misdiagnosis

Misdiagnoses occur within AIDS and within breast cancer. An HIV/AIDS misdiagnosis in women occurs most commonly in two situations. The first scenario is caused by the official CDC definition of HIV/AIDS, which was modeled after men. Second, the perception of HIV as a male condition, as well as some physicians' familiarity with male signs of HIV infection causes them to miss it in women or simply not to look for it at all.[6] In 1988, Chris Norwood highlighted the fact that women with HIV/AIDS are undercounted by the CDC. Norwood was able to show that there was an increase in women's deaths from certain infectious diseases that are most likely AIDS related. In the communities hit hardest by AIDS, women's mortality due to certain infectious diseases increased for unaccounted reasons, whereas in communities that had low AIDS rates, a similar increase in mortality due to infectious diseases was not found. These women died without ever having been diagnosed with AIDS or counted as AIDS deaths.[7] Currently, researchers still suspect that women's HIV infection is diagnosed at a later stage compared to men's, which puts these women at a disadvantage in that they receive belated secondary prevention through antiviral and prophylactic treatment.[8]

The most fundamental difference between a misdiagnosis of breast cancer and a misdiagnosis or late diagnosis of HIV is that there is no blood test that detects cancer the way the HIV antibody test determines seropositivity.[9] For cancer, three screening methods exist for the disease (breast self-exam, breast exam by a physician, and mammography). But screening for a disease is significantly different from having the means of preventing it in the first place. Further, screening is less effective and reliable than a standardized test, such as the HIV-antibody test, at predicting disease prevalence. The American Cancer Society states that the sensitivity of mammograms is between 76 percent and 94 percent, which means that in 100 women with breast cancer, mammograms miss the cancer in a minimum of 6 women to a maximum of twenty-four women. These false negatives are even higher among women younger than fifty (25 percent of cancers will be missed in this group).[10] Clinical breast exams' specificity is even lower, between 57 percent and 70 percent. In women without breast cancer, mammograms provide correct results 90 percent of the time.[11] Nevertheless, it must be noted that screening is the only available means at the present time to detect the existence of breast cancer and to thereby open the possibility for a treatment that will positively affect survival time.

Mammography is the screening method predominantly promoted by the so-called cancer establishment,[12] whose promotional campaign misrepresents mammography as a test-like procedure that definitively detects who has cancer and who is cancer free. Such misrepresentation angers cancer activists, since it alludes to a false sense of security by making women believe that mammography is a preventative measure, despite the fact that it obviously detects only what is already there. Furthermore, by the time mammography detects a cancerous lump, it has already been there for six to eight years. More important, mammography is highly imperfect; it can yield a false negative result, which can give women a false sense of security and make them believe that they have no cancer because their cancerous cells were missed in the mammogram.[13] An additional problem with this screening procedure is that mammograms are also sometimes read incorrectly by radiologists or are of such poor quality that women are erroneously told that there are no cancerous cells. Again, since there is no test that determines the existence or nonexistence of cancer, a misdiagnosis of breast cancer can also occur in other scenarios. For instance, when a woman sees a doctor because she detects or experiences a change in her breast, the doctor tells her that nothing is wrong.

Being misdiagnosed or receiving a late diagnosis adds to the new self-identity of a woman with *a disease*. Misdiagnosis is a motivational factor for women with HIV and for women with cancer. Women who are misdiagnosed are angry, and they turn their anger into activism, but the misdiagnoses are played out differently within an AIDS or a breast cancer context.

Women with misdiagnosed cancer respond with anger. Their anger stems from getting sick, even though they followed society's rules. These women believed in and supported a medical system that failed them (e.g., women who had health insurance and who acted responsibly by seeking preventative checkups). When they were diagnosed too late or misdiagnosed despite these efforts, these women responded with anger. This type of anger reflected their position of being integrated in society, and it is different than the anger of women activists with HIV.

Women activists with HIV, on the other hand, often come from situations of neglect. For instance, these women have never had health insurance and have not experienced preventative health care. Their anger reflects their specific social location outside of a system that has never served them. They consider HIV or AIDS as just one more issue on an already long list of grievances and threats to their survival. Again, this highlights the differences in race and socioeconomic status that exist between women activists with cancer and women activists with HIV.

To exemplify the differences, compare the accounts of women who have been misdiagnosed with cancer or HIV/AIDS. These two groups put their experiences with and reactions to their misdiagnoses in completely different contexts. A woman with breast cancer recalls her diagnosis:

> I went into the breast clinic in 1991. I found out that the quality of my [previous] mammograms was so poor that even if there was something there, you would never have found it and these were passed off as being acceptable by the prior radiologist. I had no idea. So that made me angry. They told me that I had this lump for 8 to 10 years. I said, "How? I had 2 mammograms, I go for my GYN visit every year. How is it that no one caught it until I found it in the shower that morning?" . . . I thought everything I was doing was right. Then you get diagnosed and like what the hell happened? And that makes you really angry, it really does. So is it what I am eating? Is it sitting in front of a computer screen? . . . That's what made me angry. I felt like I did all the right stuff. I eat vegetables, I have a fairly good diet. . . . [O]n the whole, I didn't

> feel like I had neglected myself. . . . I just didn't know what
> had gone wrong and that's what makes you mad, it really
> does. You have trust in the medical system that now I realize
> you have to take over for your own care. [cancer movement,
> with breast cancer]

This woman has expressed her frustration about not having had any
means to prevent cancer, even though she had spent considerable effort
on being a responsible, health-conscious person. Misdiagnosis trig-
gers, in the case of cancer, a sense of anger that evolves from having
done everything "right."

Women with HIV who have been misdiagnosed or diagnosed late
understand this occurrence within the context of the sexism, racism,
classism, and neglect of the medical system:

> Many women early on and still now are being misdiagnosed
> because of the definition of the opportunistic infections. They
> are not looking at that. So they are mistreated, misdiagnosed,
> oftentime not treated or then once a physician finds out that
> a person is HIV, oh it's HIV-related, you know. That's not
> gonna work. . . . It took me many months to be diagnosed
> because I didn't fit the criteria. . . . They would [not] even
> consider me to be in a category that I may be HIV infected. . . . I
> had some pretty invasive procedures for the process of elimi-
> nation [she went to the doctor with health problems] until I
> said, "Well, should you not test me for HIV?"
> *Interviewer:* So you had to bring that up?
> Oh, yeah. Definitely. And then it was a question of oh, my
> goodness. You know, like you don't have any of the other
> things. They started looking at me as a specimen. To see what's
> gonna manifest and what's gonna go on. [AIDS movement,
> tested HIV-positive nine years ago]

This account of a seropositive woman shows that her misdiagnosis
was caused by the neglect she experienced and that women still experience because of a disease that was constructed as a male disease and
consequently studied in men.

A well-known and gross example is the case of Elizabeth Ramos,
of Boston, who filed a lawsuit against Harvard Community Health
Plan for misdiagnosing her. When Ramos kept seeking medical help
from her health care providers, the providers' response was to send
her for "psychiatric help."[14]

Misdiagnosis, therefore, entails both similarities and differences between AIDS and breast cancer. One similarity is that women react with anger to their misdiagnosis and turn to activism. One difference is that these women's anger is rooted in different social locations. Prior to their diagnoses, breast cancer activists had experienced society—in particular, the medical system—as an institution that served and provided them with guidelines that, if followed, allowed them to stay healthy. On the contrary, seropositive AIDS activists had never experienced societal institutions such as the medical system as being helping, caring, or empowering. Both groups of women, however, shared that their misdiagnoses occurred because they had not been taken seriously by medical professionals when they expressed health concerns.[15]

My overall argument about mobilization combines a personal and a political relationship to the disease. Obviously, women who turn to activism after a misdiagnosis experience the disease on a daily basis, hence their personal relationship to the disease is immediate and changes their self-identity.

Misdiagnosis can remain a personal or an individualistic event in women's lives, and many misdiagnoses lead to personal reactions and individual changes. The women who turned to activism obviously went beyond personal reactions and changes. These women linked their changed self-identity to a political response. Their personal experience, misdiagnosis, became reframed into an issue of injustice. Misdiagnosis moved beyond an individual frame that explains it as a mistake made by a doctor that caused horrible personal damage to individual women's lives.

Several possible scenarios encouraged the shift from the individual occurrence to a broader matter of injustice. With regard to the specific AIDS and cancer activists I interviewed, others had already prepared or created the grounds of a collective response to the disease. AIDS organizations and grassroots cancer organizations were already in place. For instance, women with HIV were able to connect with an already existing network of AIDS organizations, which provided a political framing of what the disease meant for women.

Women who have been misdiagnosed and who have no experience of political activism connect to already existing grassroots organizations. While this explains the specific conditions that led to an involvement of my respondents at a time when organizational responses to both diseases were already in place, one questions whether misdiagnosis is a condition that has merely mobilizing potential when others have already successfully politicized the diseases. I argue that misdiagnosis is a motivational condition, whether or not grassroots organizations exist that frame the disease. However, I admit that misdiagnosis did not have the strongest *collective* mobilizing potential prior to grassroots organizations.

My overall argument that two requirements have to be present for activism, a personal and a political relationship to the disease, still applies to a misdiagnosis prior to the existence of grassroots organizations. This can be clarified in Sandra Butler's and Barbara Rosenblum's book *Cancer in Two Voices*. Rosenblum was initially misdiagnosed. In February 1985, her breast cancer was finally discovered when her prognosis was already terminal, and she died 3 years later. Hence, her diagnosis was made prior to a grassroots activist response to cancer. But she and Butler, her partner, brought their personal political history as activists to the disease. They wrote a book as a political response to breast cancer, because Rosenblum knew that "statistically she was only the first"[16] of many more women to come. She also filed a malpractice suit to heighten political awareness. She wrote in September 1985, "I know there is a point, an important point to this fight. It's about women's bodies. It's a struggle to overcome negligence and incompetence."[17] Butler recalls her partner's motivations:

> The lawsuit brought to a boil what had been simmering in her. The injustice, the economics of health care, the politics of life and death. Her experience opened her to all the women who, like her, had had poor medical care, had trusted a system that was structurally and, at times, personally unresponsive to their needs. She mobilized her anger. She raised funds for the National Women's Health Network. She spoke out and joined organizations to educate and inform women. And as always she wrote. It was not just her anger now. It was about justice.[18]

This account of Rosenblum's response to her misdiagnosis prior to the existence of any grassroots cancer organizations indicates that a mobilization and a political response about misdiagnosis are still possible. Rosenblum, an experienced critical political thinker and activist, linked the personal event of having been misdiagnosed with breast cancer to her politics and became active in cancer and women's health. This supports the overall argument that mobilization around disease by women with cancer emerges from the connection of the personal and the political. This particular case of Rosenblum's response to breast cancer also indicates how one woman's actions can set a spark, preparing the ground for larger mobilization and finally leading to mass-based grassroots organizing.

It is important to know that misdiagnosis is a unique mobilizing force. It is the approach to activism that begins most personally, through the immediate experience of the disease. But women move beyond this personal and immediate level and reframe it as a broader matter of injustice.

Misdiagnosis is a mobilizing condition as soon as it is combined with a political dimension. The political dimension could be joining an activist organization, filing a malpractice suit with the intention to seek public attention, or seeking changes that benefit a larger collective good, as was done by Ramos and Rosenblum. Malpractice suits can therefore take on a political meaning when they have been filed for reasons other than gaining reparation for personal damages suffered.[19]

Diagnosis

Living with HIV or cancer is slightly different from the condition of women who have been misdiagnosed. Superficially, both groups are living with the immediate daily experience of having a disease, but they differ because the circumstances under which they found out that they were living with a disease were different. The circumstance of having been misdiagnosed, despite one's efforts to be responsible and health conscious, is a crucial and an extraordinary ("abnormal") component of the transition from self-identity "before the disease" to a different identity "after the diagnosis." Due to these exceptional circumstances, I distinguish this group of women from women whose transition from an identity "before the disease" to a different identity "after the diagnosis" took an ordinary ("normal") course.

As I have pointed out, the diseases themselves as well as the activists who live with one or the other disease are also dissimilar. I do not mean to imply that living with a disease is the "great equalizer" between women or between diseases. In fact, living with a disease varies considerably with regard to the particularities of one's disease and factors such as race, class, and sexual orientation. These identities determine women's lives before, after, and during the new identity of living with a life-threatening illness emerges.

Women who share the identity-changing event of having tested HIV-positive or having been diagnosed with cancer are frequently novices to political activism.[20] These women's diagnoses were a trigger for their activism, and the goal of activism by first-time activists who live with the disease is to prevent others from getting the disease.

A difference between these women emerges when they name the "others" on whose behalf they are active. "Others" are those who are supposed to be spared from the disease. While it is true that the "others" are a community to which the women belong and with whom they identify, this classification is different from a community focus, which I cover in Section 4.2. First-time activists develop a community focus after they have the personal experience of being diagnosed, which is different from women who are active on behalf of their community with or without having been diagnosed.

Between first-time AIDS and cancer activists, the category of "others" has differed, because women activists with HIV/AIDS have different class and racial identities than do women cancer activists. Whereas the HIV-positive activists stem from definable oppressed communities such as substance abusers, prostitutes, and communities of color, first-time cancer activists stem from the dominant culture. Cancer activists' "others" for whom they are seeking prevention are usually women younger than themselves but similar in their class and race makeup. Often a woman within the cancer activist momement refers to daughters, nieces, or even just younger women with whom a woman identifies because she sees them as her successors. An example for such a motivational trigger is the story of a woman who identifies as a mother. She was never politically active prior to her breast cancer diagnosis, and her focus was on combining having a family, raising children, and pursuing a career.

> Since I had two young kids when I was diagnosed, I was just very focused on getting on with my life and trying to put my life back together, trying to get back into my practice, trying to figure out how I was gonna live the rest of my life and how I was gonna make sure that I was alive to be a mother to my children. And then that experience at the rally [she attended a breast cancer rally] really took me somewhat out of myself and my focus on trying to figure out how to live after breast cancer, as though there were clearly an after and though weren't an ongoing horror. So that rally took me out of that feeling and more made me aware that this was something that my daughters were going to be vulnerable to. And that so many women my age and even younger were falling prey to and

that I couldn't put my head into the sand and just trying to figure out how to get on with my own life and be a mother to my children. That I couldn't be a mother to my children unless I tried to do something about this epidemic which my children would be vulnerable to. It was at that point that I became active. [cancer movement, white, straight, with breast cancer]

These "others" include her immediate blood relatives and her children and extend from there to the larger group of her children's generation. Her "others" are the next generation of women. Hence, first-time cancer activists target a community broadly defined by gender.

Closeness and identification apply as well, according to one mother who lives with HIV. But her naming of those she wants to prevent from becoming infected reveals more than the broad community defined by gender.

I first got into this outreach, advocacy, you know, literate in that field about 3½ years ago. In the beginning, my dream was to be a voice for the many communities that I consider myself to belong to.

Interviewer: What are they?

Mm, a voice for the ex-offenders, a voice for mothers who have been incarcerated, a voice for HIV-positive mothers, a voice for lesbians, a voice for HIV-positive lesbians, a voice for people that are actively using drugs and people who are in recovery. I mean, I have lived with and in so many communities that it's hard to be a voice for one and not be a voice for the other. [AIDS movement, woman of color, lesbian, HIV-positive]

The communities to which this woman belongs reveal how different the targeted communities are between AIDS and cancer activists.

These women activists both are mothers and seek to prevent the disease in the communities to which they feel closest. That a woman prefers to define her activism in community terms rather than in family terms can be independent from whether the woman is a mother. The following quote by a mother who lives with HIV exemplifies this point:

When I went into treatment in '86 and got really on top of my life and changed my life around abusing alcohol and stuff, while I was in there, while I was in the drug treatment, I decided I needed to get back to the communities. Not that I was taken from the community, but I wanted to do something productive and a way of like giving back was to do some volunteer work. And I volunteered mainly because a friend of mine was doing some outreach in the communities, giving out "works," like paraphernalia for IV-drug users, bleach and all that stuff and talking about safer sex by using condoms, whatever. I guess I wanted to educate myself as well because I had 2 years, actually 2 years prior to doing volunteer work I was diagnosed with HIV. So that was a way for me to educate myself too. So I was going into the communities with my friends and just really doing some work. And I realized there is a lot of people out here who don't really know about that stuff. [AIDS movement, woman of color, lesbian, HIV-positive]

This woman's account reveals that her activism has been predominantly driven by a motivation to educate her former peers, the IV-drug-using community. However, the language she uses when referring to "communities," as well as other information she shared during the interview, indicates that her prevention strategy is also broader and stems from her various identities such as race and sexual orientation.

This discussion points to one important difference between first-time activists with HIV/AIDS and first-time activists with cancer. The AIDS activists seek to prevent the further spread of the disease within their disenfranchised communities, whereas the cancer activists are much more likely motivated by preventing a spread to a community that is defined solely by its gender status.

One might wish to dispute this point by insisting that first-time cancer activists' prevention strategy is actually inclusive of all of the specific communities that the HIV/AIDS activists mentioned. Breast cancer activists' focus on future generations of women can be said to include all women.[21] This is an important discussion that I cover in later chapters that look at the collective identity around gender and sexuality within AIDS and cancer activism. The later discussion focuses on the degree of inclusion that exists when one talks generically about women.

As mentioned before, women AIDS activists stem from and identify with disenfranchised communities or communities defined by multiple oppressions. This background frequently shapes these women's analysis and understanding of power. Even though the women AIDS activists are new to what is commonly recognized as political or social activism, they bring to their activism a political framework or power analysis that likens them more to women with activist experience. Various situations in their lives have prevented these women from acting on their existing consciousness about power earlier in their lives (i.e. prior to their seropositivity). Such preventive life situations include abusive relationships and drug habits. For the following woman, gender oppression in her home country functioned as such an obstacle:

> What drew me [to AIDS activism] maybe anyway even if I don't have HIV was that I grew up with a family. And in my culture, especially the women, are to be at home and take care of the kids but would never be involved with politics or outside the house. And since I was a little girl, I had to take care of myself, you know. And I always behaved different from the other women or other children. They called me like "tomboy" and comments, you know, that I tried to behave like a man, you know. . . . I was very rebelled. And when I came to the United States and saw that women can do so many things even other people don't like, you know, but they can do it, there is nothing wrong, I start to open my heart and my mind, you know. And when I came this last time, I decided to come back to school and try to develop all I can because I love what I am doing. Try to grow as a woman, break all the barriers that is around woman, nothing you can't when you can, and also help other women in the same situation. . . .
>
> *Interviewer:* Was your main reason that you found out you are HIV-positive?
>
> Not really, it was the situation about power, you know. I want to have equal opportunity, you know as a man. And here you had that option to fight back and I fought back. [AIDS movement, HIV-positive]

This keen awareness about power relationships distinguishes the first-time women AIDS activists from many first-time cancer activists who lack an understanding of oppression based on race, class, sexual orientation and, at times, even gender. Such lack of understanding of various forms of oppression stems from the first-time cancer activists' background—white, middle class, and straight—that shaped their life experiences differently from disenfranchised women with HIV.

In addition to the racial, socioeconomic, and sexual identity differences between these two groups of women, one also can find similarities. Both groups of women had been involved in life situations that hindered them from being active prior to seropositivity or cancer diagnosis. Women who had not been politically active prior to their cancer diagnosis may have chosen not to do so because they were focused on careers or on juggling a two-career family with children. The HIV-positive first-time activists are more likely to have had a consciousness about power and their social location within society, but they also were inactive prior to their seropositivity. Granted, the life situations, such as abusive relationships, drug habits, and poverty, which hindered HIV-positive women from becoming active earlier in their lives, are different obstacles than the hindrances of first-time cancer activists. First-time cancer activists' obstacles are careers, economic and social success, family responsibilities, and the like.

It has been shown that first-time activists in cancer and AIDS share a strong motivation to prevent the diseases from spreading to others. I argue that these women are active for reasons other than self-interest. Actually it appears as though these activists are the least concerned with their own survival, contradicting assumptions about self-interested motivations.

By the time women with a disease have become activists, they have reconciled their diagnoses. They hold little or no hope that activism will provide them with a personal gain for their own lives. For instance, one cancer activist states:

> No, I don't know if I think that even the fastest-moving movement is gonna do that much for me. I don't think I ever thought that in the beginning. You know that it is gonna come up other than I was gonna help to figure out how to turn metastases around if I got metastases or anything. I hoped that there would, you know that there would be some ways they could extend life a little. No, I think I thought more for the next generation . . . and I don't even know if it was that as much as just that I wanted to have the truth come out. [cancer movement, with breast cancer]

Being motivated to activism in order to prevent something from occurring within one's own community is a political act. Therefore, these women fulfill the two requirements for activism. Given that they are living with the disease, they start out with the personal relationship and then develop a political relationship by recognizing themselves as members of certain communities that they are trying to spare from the further spread of the epidemic.

SECTION 4.2 COMMUNITY ACTIVISM

In the previous section, I discussed disease prevention in communities by first-time activists who are living with diseases. However, this is different from a second mobilizing type that I discuss here, that is, preventing the further spread of the disease in one's community by community activists. The reason for differentiating between these two mobilizing conditions is that community activists are cognizant of their community membership, regardless of health status. Community activists are women whose personal identity overlaps with the collective identity of their community. On the other hand, first-time activists developed a community focus after they experienced changes in their personal identity due to a diagnosis.

Before proceeding with this discussion, I will define what I mean here by "community." I define community as a counter-cultural group of individuals that is smaller than society. Group members share a collective identity that reflects and affirms the members' common interests that run counter to the dominant culture's norms and values. This definition is different from a social movement "community," which is essentially a politically motivated and derived formation of collective action that can be independent of the participants' personal identities. This form of politically motivated activism is covered in the next section as the political approach. This section, however, covers women who are active on behalf of the communities of color and lesbian communities. While women who are motivated by prevention for their communities live with and without the disease, they also belong to the communities on whose behalf they are active.

It is important to recall the differences between the diseases themselves. AIDS has known ways of transmission, which makes the disease preventable and therefore controllable, whereas we are less certain about the causes of breast cancer.[22] This difference leads to different conditions for mobilization. Whereas AIDS activists can reach out to their communities and educate in order to prevent others from contracting HIV, cancer activists' means of prevention are more indirect. Cancer activism and mobilization for prevention depend on influencing authorities and other powers to take action to find causes and ban the usage of substances known to cause cancer.

Within AIDS activism, one finds a number of programs that target specific communities for prevention. For instance, one highly effective model, peer education, directly targets certain communities and is put into action by women who are living with HIV/AIDS.

Women of Color

In this section I discuss women of color activists within AIDS or cancer activism who usually are without the disease but often have professional skills that bring them to these movements. Coming to activism through one's professional skills, combined with community focus, is the most common motivation for women of color. That women of color often become involved in this manner is an important factor that has been historically acknowledged for African-American women. Patricia Hill Collins uses the term *community othermother* to describe this form of political activism, which she sees as the foundation for "Black women's political activism."[23] Community othermothers have a crucial role within the African-American community because they work on sustaining and further developing the community:

> Black women's involvement in fostering African-American community development forms the basis for community-based power. This is the type of power many African Americans have in mind when they describe the 'strong Black women' they see around them in traditional African-American communities. Community othermothers work on behalf of the Black community by expressing ethics of caring and personal accountability which embrace concepts of transformative power and mutuality (Kuykendall 1983). Such power is transformative in that Black women's relationships with children and *other vulnerable community members* is not intended to dominate or control. Rather, its purpose is to bring people along, to—in the words of late-nineteenth-century Black feminists— "uplift the race" so that *vulnerable members* of the community will be able to attain the self-reliance and independence essential for resistance. [emphasis added][24]

This concept of community othermothers can be applied to the position of many women of color activists who are without either disease. As vulnerable community members, one can envision women with a disease or at risk of contracting one. Whereas Collins and bell hooks[25] refer to professionals such as teachers, my purpose is to apply the term *community othermother* to health care providers who serve, educate, and advocate for their communities.

The existence of this historically female version of political activism, acting as community othermothers, also explains women's motivations and indicates the organizational type that will be developed. These organizations will be created by community othermothers and will be community-based organizations. This is contrary to the emergence of cancer grassroots organizations, which are mostly an outcome of activism by white women with cancer. One of the women of color cancer activists I interviewed addressed this racial difference between cancer activists directly when she stated:

> This is a conference that's called, "Breast Cancer: Nurses as Change Agents." And all these people here, I can't speak for this person, everyone else is a person of color. So maybe from these kind of programs there will be kind of like an uprising. But the interesting thing is that the process is still different. For example, if you look at the grassroots organizations they were from women that suffer from breast cancer themselves. But looking on the minority front, it seems like it's from the women that are service providers. Because I can't speak for all African-American women but just that a disproportionate number of us are poor, have no insurance. It seems like the service providers are uprising and organizing something versus the women who are impacted by breast cancer themselves. And this goes back to before, and this is like the worst case, because we are all not poor. But if you are poor you are on welfare, you have kids, you have no daycare and everything else and then you have to run back and forth to chemotherapy, if you even have time to do that. You don't have time to organize a movement around breast cancer. [cancer movement, woman of color, without cancer]

Her argument illuminates some of the differences that exist between cancer activists in terms of racial background. Moreover, women's racial identities also create different realities and motivations for activism.

Professional motivations apply to AIDS activists without the disease as well, and many of the women of color take a similar position to HIV/AIDS than women of color cancer activists:

> I think that coming from a background of the voice of the
> voiceless. I think that our communities are, right now I am
> speaking from the Latino community, because immigration
> laws are the laws for aliens that come from other places. A lot
> of people are not benefiting from the services that they could
> get. I feel that because I am an educated woman and because
> I care for the community, I can help in that situation. I can be
> a voice but although be the one that can work with the com-
> munity, inform them what are their rights and in terms of HIV
> and AIDS. . . . I think that I didn't become involved into this
> work because I was at risk, but I thought that my community
> is at risk. And that is what moved me to do something. [AIDS
> movement, woman of color, HIV-negative]

All of the previously mentioned or quoted women activists are women
of color and articulate the motivation for their activism in similar
ways. It is a combination of having the professional skills and caring
deeply for their communities.

It is important to discuss professionally motivated and commu-
nity-oriented activists in the context of the general argument that
women's activism stems from having a personal and a political relationship to the disease. Some of the women who come to activism
through a professional motivation appear to contradict this argument,
because they do not necessarily have a personal relationship to the
disease when they start their work.

Generally a personal relationship to the disease consists of two
alternatives. Either the woman has the disease herself or someone to
whom she feels close is diagnosed with cancer or tests HIV-positive.
As I mentioned, the professional women are generally HIV-negative
or without cancer. Moreover, many of these professional women did
not have someone in their lives who was living with either disease
when they started their work. This could dispute my general argument, that there is always a personal and political relationship for
women who turn to activism, however, I offer a different explanation
for this seeming inconsistency.

I argue that women of color activists who come to activism through
a professional or community involvement nevertheless have a personal relationship to the disease. I draw on the introduced concept of
the *community othermother*, which I suggested as the fitting term for
this type of activism. A community othermother's relationship to her
community is nothing other than personal, because she is rooted in

and deeply connected to her community. The concept of *community othermother* "models a very different value system, one whereby Afrocentric feminist ethics of caring and personal accountability move communities forward."[26] Hence a personal relationship exists, even though it might not follow the common understanding of personal tie that I put forward earlier and defined as knowing and being close to an individual. A community othermother knows and is close to the vulnerable members of her community, even though, prior to her activism, she might not always have personally known individuals living with cancer or AIDS.

White women with professional skills are also motivated by prevention of the disease in their communities. I have decided not to discuss this in more detail here, because the white women who have professional skills and community motivation are usually lesbians, whose perspective is discussed in the following section. Straight white women who come to activism because of "community prevention" generally have the disease themselves, and their case is also discussed separately. Apart from these groups, I found very few exceptions of straight white women who are without disease, have professional skills, and are motivated by prevention for their communities. These women's understanding of prevention is different, because it applies to future generations instead of to prevention for communities. Defining prevention broadly, for the benefit of future generations, is different from the specific focus of community activists. Women of color and lesbians stem from and are active within definable communities, whereas a white straight woman without the disease who is active to prevent the disease for future generations refers to nothing other than the dominant society.

Lesbians

Most of the lesbians within both movements have a background in political activism. The lesbians who contradict this claim and were mobilized without prior political experience are HIV-positive lesbians who are first-time activists, as discussed earlier.

Lesbians' motivations for activism primarily reflect a desire to be active in their communities.[27] The communities with which lesbians identify are the gay and lesbian community or the feminist community, stemming from their self-identity as *women*.

The lesbians whom I interviewed placed their activism in these movements within the context of prior political activism within the gay and lesbian movement or the women's movement. Furthermore, many of my respondents claimed that lesbians have a heightened political awareness. One activist involved in many political movements and social change activities explained:

> Lesbians have been the fucking shock troops for every social issue since I have been a lesbian. . . . In the early 80s when everybody was sort of lying down in the streets and doing all this Central America activism . . . a lot of lesbians were involved in that. A lot of lesbians were involved in abortion rights and you know, we don't need abortions. We have been, I think, I don't know why this is, and this is probably a central question, we have been really capable of looking at a big picture, feminist issues, and discovering this sort of underlying way to be activist. [AIDS movement]

That a high level of politicization among lesbians is common has been confirmed by other researchers who investigated lesbian involvement in AIDS. Melissa McNeill reported that fourteen out of the nineteen lesbians she interviewed who are involved in AIDS work had prior involvement in political causes or social change movements.[28] Similarly, Nancy Stoller argues that, beginning in the early 1980s, the lesbians who entered the AIDS epidemic have been influenced by the culture created during the 1970s by the women's movement and the gay and lesbian movement. Furthermore, Stoller points out that as the 1980s began, women (including lesbians) were occupationally located to encounter men with HIV due to their dominance as health providers, social workers, and health educators.[29] According to Stoller, this created the situation that lesbians were involved in two ways: not only as professionals, but also as women (feminists) and as lesbians—"two potential master statuses"[30] that affected the roles lesbians played in the AIDS epidemic.

Stoller's argument points to the three motivational conditions that encourage lesbians to become involved in the AIDS movement. First, lesbians are professionally situated so they come into contact with people with HIV. Second, they are involved as women who act on a feminist consciousness. Third, they act on their membership within the gay and lesbian community. Whether these three motivational conditions are different among AIDS and cancer activists is discussed later.

Stoller's "two master statuses" (woman/feminist and lesbian) plus professional status motivate lesbians who moved into AIDS activism early. This is evident in the following account of a lesbian AIDS activist, reminiscing about her motivational reasons in the early 1980s:

> At that point, I was the head of the gay nurses alliance, which was an international group that no longer exists, and through that group I knew a lot of people from different parts of the United States and Canada. And we started to hear strange things coming out of a lot of different emergency rooms about this new disease. And then in '81–'82 the media began to pick it up. . . . It was sort of natural that I would move into the area where my brothers and sisters, my brothers most of the time, were dying. [AIDS movement]

The gay and lesbian community was a strong motivational factor, especially among early AIDS activists. In fact, many of these activists were criticized in the 1980s for their gay and lesbian community focus. The theoretical position from which these attacks were made was radical feminism or lesbian separatism, which shared a rejection of putting energy into men. One of the most vocal critics of lesbians' AIDS activism has been radical feminist Sonia Johnson, who argued against lesbian involvement, even in the late 1980s.[31]

> [Lesbians] can also give much time and energy to AIDS work to find again that our efforts are taken for granted and, worst of all, that we have no time left for our own work, for women's revolution. Because history attests that there will always be some urgent reason, such as AIDS, for women to put aside our important concerns, we must insist now on putting our own lives first, we must refuse to get sidetracked again. Abolition sidetracked us, the peace movement sidetracked us, Central American politics and the so-called New Age movement have currently united with AIDS to sidetrack us. We can go on forever fighting men's battles.[32]

Lesbian AIDS activists are familiar with these criticisms and have responded to them many times during the 1980s and even more recently, although AIDS is no longer perceived as a "gay male" disease.

Gay and lesbian community focus among AIDS activists

The lesbians responding to such criticisms highlight various points. Lesbians readily admit that their motivation to be active in AIDS, at a time when it was defined as a gay male disease, is not something that gay men would have chosen to do for lesbians had the disease emerged in the lesbian population. A unanimous voice emerged among lesbians that, had AIDS emerged among lesbians first, we would all be dead by now. Nevertheless, this common belief among lesbians is generally independent of lesbians' motivations toward AIDS activism. Lesbians argue that their motivation to become active must not be misconstrued as helping others only if they are willing to reciprocate. "[T]hat's not why I am [an AIDS activist], so somebody will take care of me if I get a fatal disease. It's about solidarity" [AIDS movement]. Thus, we see solidarity as a motivating factor. The solidarity to which lesbians are referring is rooted in their sense of belonging to one community—here the gay and lesbian community.

> [H]ow could we have done anything else? Even if it had turned out to be only a gay men's disease for ever and ever, there still would be a certain number of us and other people who should have been saying this is unconscionable, these people are suffering, let me see what I can do. Because that is a real human response. It is a response from a place that wants to create healing and compassion in the world. To me I hope there are some lesbian women running around talking about they want to help. I think *we would be a much poorer community* if we didn't have people who have had that authority of compassionate response and even forgiveness sort of tied to it. [AIDS movement] [emphasis added]

Therefore, a focus on the gay and lesbian community is one motivational factor that brought lesbians into AIDS activism, especially in the early years prior to the recognition of AIDS as a disease that also affected women.

Moreover, gay and lesbian community focus is a prominent motivational factor among lesbians who perceived the lack of the government's response as rooted within homophobia. These women defined homophobia as a hatred against the gay and *lesbian* community.[33] The gay and lesbian community became more visible in the 1980s due to the AIDS epidemic. Therefore, lesbians who were motivated by a community focus made a link between their self-identity and the conditions and future of their community, especially since lesbians knew that they would also suffer from the increase in homophobia that was caused by the emergence of the AIDS crisis. Mainstream society does not distinguish lesbians from gay men. This motivation is similar for women of color who become active on behalf of their community due to their racial identity.

Feminist community focus within AIDS

Many lesbians have entered AIDS activism with a feminist consciousness and experiences stemming from their involvement in the women's movement. This applies both to early AIDS activists and to lesbians who joined AIDS activism later. Due to their feminist consciousness, many lesbians are credited with bringing women into conversations about AIDS. The motivational perspective of these lesbians who are in solidarity with women has been frequently neglected whenever lesbians' motivations are discussed. Failure to mention this fact creates a misperception of lesbians' motivations; presenting lesbians as though they are solely motivated by a solidarity to gay men shortchanges their motivations. Some lesbians have been motivated by solidarity with *women*. Other lesbians argue that they responded with a gay and lesbian community focus because they anticipated a backlash against their community that would include lesbians.

The reasoning and participation of lesbians is a neglected aspect of AIDS activism, hence women with AIDS or at risk for HIV and the women activists themselves fall prey to sexism and secondary status. I make no claim that solidarity with gay men has been the primary motivation for lesbians, and solidarity with women due to a feminist consciousness became a secondary motivation among lesbians only at a later time.[34] Instead it is important to note that lesbian AIDS activists have cited both motivational factors. Hence I claim that presenting lesbians' motivations as a single approach—their sole motivation is solidarity with gay men—is a misconstruction of the complexity of their motivations.

The lesbians I interviewed point to a multitude of motivating facts. For instance, many of them encountered women with HIV early on in the epidemic. Gender bias and homophobia led to the assumption that AIDS was a gay male disease, but many of my lesbian respondents argued that they were aware that a sexually transmitted disease does not stay within one segment of the population as the health authorities would have the public believe.

Most certainly we have learned from the AIDS epidemic that we need to make a distinction between sexual identity and sexual practice. One's identity is not a predictor of one's sexual practice. The lines are much more blurred than previously believed or defined by societal institutions such as the CDC. Studies have shown that "lesbians" have sex with men, "gay men" have sex with women, and "heterosexual husbands" contracted HIV while engaging in male-to-male sex. According to the CDC, a lesbian is a woman who has had sexual relations exclusively with females from 1977 until her AIDS diagnosis. "This excludes the *majority* of women who have sex with women and or define themselves as lesbians"[35] [emphasis added]. Instead we know that more women have sex with women than self-identify as lesbians.[36] In reality, lesbians make a variety of choices in terms of practices and behaviors. Some use IV drugs and others sell sex to men for money or in exchange for drugs. Of course, the same is also true for other sexual identities. For instance, a study of gay men in New York City showed that "72 percent of 205 respondents had had female sexual partners at some time in their lives, the median number between three and four per man."[37]

Awareness about women and AIDS and women's risks of contracting HIV has been politicized and voiced by lesbians involved in AIDS activism. Others admit that it was frequently lesbian leadership that pushed AIDS organizations or the public to recognize the needs of HIV-infected women. For instance, Carol Glassman argues that the lesbian members of AIDS organizations pushed the National Institutes of Health to establish a special women's section within their institutional AIDS response team.[38] This indicates that lesbians have been active on behalf of women. The connection between lesbians' feminist identity and their location within the community of women, a community defined by sharing a gender status, is one motivational factor that moved lesbians to AIDS activism. One activist argued:

> [O]verwhelmingly, this is becoming a disease of women and particularly those of us who are lesbians. Part of what that means is that we love women, okay. And so even if the women that are infected by this disease only some of them are lesbians, others of them have orientations of various other persuasions, they are still people of whom we have tried to create a different world environment. [AIDS movement]

Feminist community focus within cancer

Solidarity is one motivation that has brought lesbians into AIDS activism. Is this motivation identical with feminist-motivated breast cancer activism? This is indeed the case. Most lesbians within cancer activism argue that they have been motivated by understanding cancer as a women's issue, just as lesbians within AIDS understand AIDS as a women's issue. Lesbians within cancer activism embrace their self-identity as women and connect to the larger community of women. Having pointed out similarities in motivational approaches, however, it is also important to point to the differences that exist between the two approaches.

Differences in lesbian-feminist motivations

The two motivational approaches are only identical in that they are rooted within a feminist consciousness. But lesbian activists motivated by feminism are affected differently by the outcome and success of AIDS and cancer activism. Whereas lesbian activists within AIDS are generally HIV-negative and perceive themselves as active on behalf of other women, this is not the case with cancer.[39] The lesbians within cancer activism motivated by feminism are those both with and without cancer. When one compares lesbians without cancer to lesbian HIV-negative AIDS activists, the likelihood of developing cancer is perceived as higher than the likelihood of contracting HIV. Therefore, the motivation of lesbians to become active on behalf of women and cancer can be perceived as being much closer to self-interest, even though any given lesbian activist may be cancer free. Such potential self-interest can be seen in the account of a lesbian who has never had cancer. She begins by clarifying her feminist motivations for activism. For her, cancer is a gender parity issue. Following this belief, she points out that she perceives herself as being potentially at risk:

> [B]reast cancer is a really good example of the disparity in research dollars between men and women. And that is one of the things that for me is so critical to us fighting for the cause of breast cancer, to find out what the cause of breast cancer is so that we can prevent it, because so little of our national research dollars goes into women's health issues and it wasn't until a couple of years ago that even those percentages started

to rise. So if they were looking at heart disease, they were looking at white men. They were looking at lung cancer, colon cancer, any number of cancers, most of the cases they used were always men. . . . I see that as a really good organizing tool. It's a way of bringing attention to the fact that women's health issues need to be studied separately from the issues of men. So there are a number of levels for me where it hits me. One is on a personal level of knowing women with breast cancer, being affected by it, knowing that I am as much at risk as anybody else of getting it, of developing breast cancer. [cancer movement]

In addition to the potential for future self-interest among lesbians within cancer activism, there is another difference between the two movements. Feminism embraces cancer as a women's issue because it is seen as *the* health threat to all women. Such perception of cancer activism as the "right" cause is the mirror opposite to the criticisms lesbians in AIDS activism faced. Contrary to AIDS, cancer activism evolved among feminists as the "right" kind of activism.

Some lesbian cancer activists have cancer themselves. This marks another difference in lesbian AIDS activists. Some lesbian cancer activists with cancer actually moved from AIDS activism to cancer activism. A prominent example is Jackie Winnow. Winnow had been involved in AIDS activism and described herself as an AIDS caregiver.[40] While she was active in AIDS activism, she was diagnosed with breast cancer in 1985. In 1988, she was diagnosed with metastatic breast cancer, and she spoke out:

[A]pproximately forty thousand women were living with cancer in the San Francisco/Oakland area, at least four thousand being lesbians, about four thousand women dying. Eight thousand women were diagnosed this year. The forty thousand women don't have the services that the hundred women with AIDS have. I want the women with AIDS to have these services. I don't mean to polarize. But I also want recognition that we have a huge problem here and we need to do something about it.[41]

Winnow and other lesbians acted to bridge the gap in services and resources. In 1986, she founded the Women's Cancer Resource Center in Berkeley, California. The center provides support, information, and resources to women to empower them to make decisions about their lives.[42]

Focus on the lesbian community

In addition to lesbians who were motivated to found *women's* cancer organizations, other lesbians directed their efforts specifically to organizations for lesbians. The most well known of these organizations is the Mary-Helen Mautner Project for Lesbians with Cancer. Notably, many lesbian activists within the lesbian cancer organizations are themselves without cancer. The motivations and organizations that lesbian activists created mirror those of gay and lesbian AIDS activists, focusing on their community and providing support, advocacy, and education. This similarity is not surprising, since many of these lesbians who are involved in cancer organizations were involved with AIDS activism before cancer activism. Despite Winnow's example, not all lesbians who switch from AIDS activism to cancer activism do so due to a cancer diagnosis. Some lesbian cancer activists define their motivations as focusing specifically on the lesbian community, and other lesbians focus more broadly on the community of women. The same is true within the context of AIDS. A variety of AIDS organizations have emerged from different communities and sometimes cater to other specific communities as well. Within AIDS, there are specific women's AIDS organizations and one Lesbian AIDS Project in New York City.

Personal and political

Within this section, the motivations of lesbians are linked to lesbian self-identity and an identification with the gay and lesbian community, the women's/feminist community, or any combination of these. No consistent external factors can explain whether a lesbian chooses to have the self-identity of a lesbian over that of a woman and thereby becomes active on behalf of lesbians or women. For instance, one cannot argue that lesbians who are active on behalf of the lesbian community are "out" or "more out" than the women who are motivated by a women's community focus.

Both differences and similarities exist between lesbians within the AIDS and cancer movements. There are a number of misperceptions about differences between lesbians in the cancer movement in comparison to lesbians in the AIDS movement. Such false assumptions, for instance, argue that lesbians within AIDS are younger than lesbians within cancer, or that lesbians switched to cancer due to a cancer diagnosis, that lesbians within cancer are feminists, and that the lesbians within AIDS self-identify exclusively with their sexual orientation. I found that none of these assumptions held upon closer examination.[43]

Lesbians within AIDS and within cancer have claimed both political and personal reasons. The specific personal reasons for a lesbian's involvement vary. Overall, they are identical to the kind already discussed for various other motivational types—if someone to whom one feels close is HIV-positive, if someone to whom one feels close has cancer, or if one has cancer oneself—these are the most common personal reasons among lesbians. Additionally, as with women of color, underlying their activism on behalf of one's community is a political and a personal reason. Lesbians feel close to members of their community, whether or not they have personally known an individual with the disease before their activism. An important reminder in this context is that some women of color who have been quoted here are lesbians, and some of the quoted lesbians are women of color. The separate presentation of women of color's motivation from lesbian's motivation is artificial and should not be misread that women of color are straight and lesbians are white.

SECTION 4.3 POLITICAL-IDEOLOGICAL APPROACH

Women who are politically motivated to join the cancer or AIDS movement are not unlike women who are motivated to prevent a further spread of the disease within their communities. Being motivated by concern for one's community is a political act. Nevertheless, I distinguish community-motivated activism from what I call "political-ideological activism" for the following reasons. I have defined community-focused activism as one pursued by women whose self-identity is tied to the collective identity of a community on whose behalf one has become active. Women who identify strongly with a community with which they share a racial or a sexual identity experience their connection to other members of their community as personal, regardless of their actual familiarity with others. On the contrary, a political-ideological approach to activism is rooted in a self-identity that is more abstract and connects women to an "ideological community," which is a network of like-minded people. This applies to social movement communities as I explained earlier, such politically-

ideologically motivated communities are made up of environmental-
ists or feminists, among others. The members of these more abstract
communities are less easy to determine. For instance, whether a woman
is a feminist first has to be determined. The community focus has an
underpinning of identity and community that is experienced physically, therefore, the connection to community members is personal.
Like-mindedness or membership in a theoretically created community
has to be confirmed first, and then a personal connection to members
is possible.

This differentiation between community focus and the abstract
thought community allows us to discuss women who might even have
an oppositional identity (e.g., they are lesbians) but are motivated by
more abstract political reasons rather than concerns for their community. Furthermore, straight white, middle-class activists have been
mostly excluded from the community discussion thus far. These
women's race, class, and sexual identity are not oppositional to the
dominant culture, however, these white middle-class straight women
constitute a number of activists who have a predominant political (i.e.,
feminist) approach to activism.

This type of political-ideological approach to activism applies to
women who already have political experience by the time they enter
the arena of AIDS or breast cancer activism. What follows is a discussion of mobilization based on collective identities that women bring to
their activism.

I argue that this motivational condition is most important for many
activists within the cancer movement, whereas it is slightly less
significant within the AIDS movement. The women who fit the criterion of having a political-ideological motivation and are involved in
cancer activism are those both with and without the disease. More
succinctly, the women who found grassroots cancer organizations are
usually women who live with cancer themselves and have been involved in political activism before their cancer diagnosis.

The political-ideological approaches to cancer activism

In 1989, Susan Shapiro published an article in the feminist magazine *Sojourner* that has been instrumental for grassroots activism. It
triggered the founding of cancer organizations in the Boston area.[44]

> From the time my mother was diagnosed with breast cancer
> until she died of it eleven years later, it did not occur to me

that her illness was a feminist issue. Even my own experience of having cancer did not arouse my sense of politics. Like most people, I had learned that cancer was a personal tragedy; it was not a community issue, certainly not within the realm of feminist causes. . . . It is no wonder that feminists haven't taken on a cause that on the surface appears apolitical, hopeless, and frightening. Unlike incest, battering, discrimination, and other feminist concerns, cancer does not seem to be an issue of empowerment vs. oppression (although race, socioeconomic status, and gender certainly influence our treatment and, in some cases, survival rates). . . . Cancer is clearly a feminist issue. We need an organization—of women, for women—that will encompass political action, direct service, and education.[45]

Even though Shapiro herself had cancer, she drew predominantly on her political framework, feminism, and applied it to develop new cancer activist organizations. Political perspectives other than feminism have also been brought to the cancer movement. Women whose prominent political issues are environmental justice or women's health also shaped cancer activism.

The existing grassroots cancer organizations distribute newsletters, fact sheets, and flyers that reinforce the mobilization of women who have a political consciousness around feminism, environment, and health.[46] By putting forth these issues, mobilization occurs around a more abstract thought community that shares a collective identity with other movements such as the feminist, environment, and health movements.

These three political frameworks, or ideologies, are feminism, environment, or health, and they are the dominant issues that women bring with them to cancer activism. They are also the issues that prevail within cancer activism. A few women among the cancer activists have additional political issues than these three, however. For instance, the following seasoned activist mentioned what attracted her to cancer activism; her answer was quite different than others'.

Well, I wasn't attracted to it. I think I saw the cancer issue as more or less one of these individual things that happens to people. . . . I read Susan Shapiro's article in *Sojourner*. It was really an eye-opener to me. . . . The thing that brought me into it when I did finally come to it was the idea that there is such a discrepancy between the way that women's cancer is treated depending on their income level. So my reason for getting involved in the women's cancer movement was poor women and women not having health insurance and not getting treated. [cancer movement, with cancer]

This woman's agenda locates her, according to her own words, more on the fringes of this movement, because her issue—injustice due to income inequality or racial differences—has not been taken up by the movement. She remained part of the movement because of her personal relationship, even though she had given up on seeing her political concerns realized.

Boundaries of mobilization around cancer or AIDS

The boundaries of mobilization to cancer activism were stated earlier. Women without cancer whose main concerns are class or race analysis, similar to the woman with cancer, quoted above, are not found within the cancer movement.

Similar boundary issues can be found within AIDS activism. The dominant issues are to improve health and also to fight sexism, racism, classism, and homophobia. I also encountered a number of women AIDS activists who said that spirituality is an important motivating issue for their involvement. But as with cancer activism, women whose main concern is spirituality, with no other aspect to share with the dominant frames of AIDS activism, are not found in that movement.[47] Further, I encountered white and middle-class HIV-positive women who felt there were no appropriate activist opportunities for them, either within AIDS activism or in support groups.[48]

Differences between cancer and AIDS

Women with or without cancer join cancer activism for the political reasons mentioned earlier, hence cancer activists' health status is of no importance to this political-ideological approach to cancer activism. But this does not hold true for AIDS activists. The activists to which this political-ideological approach to AIDS activism can be applied are HIV-negative. The HIV-positive activists within AIDS have already been presented as first-time activists who enter AIDS activism with a political consciousness but with little or no experience in other social movements.

While this motivational type applies to HIV-negative activists only, not all HIV-negative activists are covered by this particular political-ideological approach; some have been discussed as being motivated by community activism.

The politically-ideologically motivated type applies predominantly to white middle-class straight women. For instance, I did not encounter any straight white women who were AIDS activists, the segment of the population most suited for this category, as shown for cancer activism.[49]

Hence the motivational type covers HIV-negative women activists who claimed that their motivation was based on something other than on behalf of their community—in other words, women who became active based on feminism, classism, or racism. Some white lesbians have offered this line of argument. They are active within the AIDS or cancer movements and argue that their motivation has been mostly or completely independent from concerns for the gay and lesbian community.

Within AIDS activism, these white lesbians can often be found in AIDS organizations that did not emerge from the gay and lesbian community. Those who analyzed the history of AIDS organizations claim that gay and lesbian community-based organizations were in place by 1985 and had achieved hegemony when public health officials finally responded.[50] AIDS organizations rooted in communities of color or those focused on women had a different course of mobilization and emerged after gay and lesbian community-based organizations were already in place.[51] One seldom-acknowledged arena is the responses by prostitutes who were active in self-empowerment and prostitute rights organizations. These women acted as AIDS peer educators for other prostitutes. Similarly, a less publicized response was AIDS education projects that emerged in prisons.[52] AIDS also formed many new communities, such as the People Living with AIDS movement (PLWA), which was launched in 1983.[53]

Some lesbians within cancer activism have been motivated for environmental and feminist reasons, therefore, they are active for the benefit of women and frame breast cancer as a women's issue caused by the environment, and by no means is a lesbian issue. These lesbians within cancer activism are working in feminist cancer organizations that frame cancer as a feminist and environmental issue. Lesbians within AIDS activism, however, who are motivated by racism, classism, and feminism, work within organizations that advocate for substance abusers, prostitutes, and the like. One white lesbian activist explained her motivation to AIDS activism with anti-racism:

I can honestly say, I was just very struck with the lack of anything going on around AIDS in this community particularly as it related to communities of color. . . . I ended up . . . starting a group of basically Cape Verdean, Latino, and African-American and white folk to really look at how this epidemic is in our community. . . . I started doing much more grassroots organizing with churches and community organizations and different people who were in recovery. Then when I met this guy . . . we really started looking much more analytically at the virus and its impact on IV-drug users in [location] because he knew a lot of people who are IV-drug users who had the virus and that was '88, '89. When we really started looking at it analytically and 38 percent of the people with AIDS in [location] were IV-drug related. And now it's twice that: 3 out of 4 people with AIDS have it as a result of IV-drug use. So the profile of the epidemic here in [location] is very different than the rest of the state and also the rest of the country. [AIDS movement, white, lesbian, HIV-negative]

The two components, personal and political

Two conditions, the personal and the political relationship, have to be present for mobilization, but a discussion of the three motivational types acknowledges differences regarding the dominance of the personal over the political relationship, and vice versa. Two arguments show how important the presence is of both components. The first becomes clear with the example of a woman who has had a political interest prior to her personal relationship with cancer. Her story highlights that a political connection alone was not enough motivation to get involved.

I sent money to them in honor of [a friend's] mother. And, then they sent me a brochure. They sent me the packet, the information about the group. And I thought, oh, this group looks really interesting. . . . I have always been interested in women's health in general. I am not a health care worker but it has just been always an interest of mine and I thought, some day when I have some time and energy, I would like to maybe get involved with this group. It sounds like they are doing really good work. And then I put it aside and aside and aside and then I went for

> my routine mammogram and they found an abnormality in my mammogram. I had a biopsy, it was malignant and then I had a mastectomy and all that. And suddenly, I mean, I heard about the [organization] and I immediately started going to meetings. So I already knew about them from somebody else and they were in the back of my mind. But once I got that diagnosis, I felt really lucky, because I knew exactly where to find them. [cancer movement, with breast cancer]

Her description shows that, until the personal aspect was present, she postponed her activism, despite the fact that the group corresponded directly to women's health, which was an important political interest of hers. The friend's mother who had died earlier had not provided her with a personal relationship to the disease because she was not close to her friend's mother. Donating money to the cancer organization merely fulfilled a friend's request. Her personal relationship to cancer was fulfilled after she was diagnosed with cancer herself. Only then did she become active.

The importance of the presence of both of these conditions is attested to by those respondents I encountered within AIDS activism who are actually living with cancer. These women have a personal relationship to cancer but choose instead to stay within AIDS activism. They choose to be active with a disease other than the one they have, for two reasons. First, AIDS activists who live with these unusual circumstances are community activists (ideal type 2) or politically-ideologically motivated activists (ideal type 3). They also have a personal relationship to AIDS. But these women's political convictions are predominantly addressed by AIDS, and breast cancer activism does not address their concerns. This is linked to the discussion of the boundaries of mobilization regarding cancer and AIDS. I stated earlier that AIDS activism centers around issues of sexism, racism, classism, and homophobia, whereas cancer activism addresses issues of sexism, health, and the environment.[54]

While both connections have to be present, the personal relationship dominates the first motivational ideal type (diagnosis), whereas the political connection dominates the third motivational type. This can also be examined by paying attention to the connections through which women enter activism. Frequently women who are predominantly motivated by a personal relationship first enter support groups or participate in programs that cater to women with the disease. The support the women experience in these settings enables them to go beyond support groups into activism. On the contrary, women who are motivated mostly due to a political connection move into activist groups right away. Given that some of these women have cancer, it is interesting that they either do not take advantage of support groups or they attend them, after they have found the political organizations to which they are drawn.

These women who live with the disease explain their motivation to activism as a connection to their personal life circumstance—for instance, having cancer with a connection to interests in politics, feminism, the environment, or health. Most women claim that this combination of personal and political is powerful; one woman called it a "Eureka experience." Making the step to involvement is seen as "natural" because it brings together aspects that had already been present separately in women's lives.

> [The triggering event is a letter to the editor in *Science for the People* magazine written by Judy Brady.[55]] I was just astonished that there was somebody else out there who was linking pesticides with cancer and who was interested in the environmental connection and I was just beginning, to think of that. . . . I needed to go abroad to be politicized and see how power works. . . . So I did all this work in Central America and Africa and became increasingly political. So I was really ready to look at cancer from that perspective. I don't think I would have done it had I not met Judy Brady, because she is the one who made me realize that my own life was also involved with this. So at that point, I was no longer just being an observer to other people's revolutions. It was about me, too. And so I could bring all parts of my self to the question . . . it was kind of like a spark. You know, it pulled everything together for me. All my political ideas, all my [environmental] ideas, and all my personal history, all came together, and it was really Judy that did it. [cancer movement, with cancer]

This woman brought her environmental consciousness to her mobilization around cancer.

A discussion of women's political concerns shows that women with a disease are not narrowly motivated to involvement by potential self-gains. Instead, they are applying their political ideas to their personal situations.

For women who do not have diseases themselves, the requirement of a personal and a political relationship also applies. For example, many women with a political history join cancer or AIDS organizations after a close friend, family member, or someone else close to them has developed cancer or has tested HIV-positive.

However, there is clearly a difference between the activists with a disease and those without. Many politically-ideologically motivated activists who are not living with a disease themselves see their activism as similar to other causes they have taken on at an earlier time in their lives.

> It feels satisfying to me the way that the pieces of my life have come together now. But I don't feel like this is significantly different than the epiphany I had around the domestic violence movement or around any other issue. There is the local organizing that happens, there is the statewide, there is the national, there is even the international. And I feel that in terms of breast cancer also. The one thing that I feel really different about is, I do feel some real hope that through organizing around breast cancer that we can really raise awareness and really make a difference. . . . So I feel like I am a part of an important movement in that sense that it has a lot of potential. No, overall I don't feel that this is drastically different than other things I have been involved in. [cancer movement, without cancer]

This indicates that, for women without disease, identifying with others has the same importance within their identity as other issues have. The individual identity of women without disease is that of activist: they care about the issue, and they care deeply about the women who have the disease, but this is comparable to other types of involvement they have experienced before. As activists, they have learned to identify with others by establishing commonalities with the identities of gender, ethnicity, race, class, and sexual orientation.

Conclusion

Three motivational approaches to cancer and AIDS have been discussed. Even though all three have been found within both AIDS and cancer activism, some of these categories are more important for one movement and less important for another. For instance, lesbians motivated by a gay and lesbian community focus are central to AIDS activism, but they are marginal within cancer activism. Among women of color, the community focus is a historically affirmed form of activism, and it is of little importance whether the organizing issue is cancer or AIDS.

All three motivational types—diagnosis, community focus, and a political-ideological approach—describe motivations to activism that entail both a personal and a political relationship to the disease. As discussed earlier, the motivational categories describe ideal motivational types. Creating such a typology produces the artificial situation of discussing women activists as though they had one identity corresponding to one motivational type. Of course, women activists' identities are in reality more complex, multilayered, and less separate than they appear throughout this discussion of motivational conditions. For instance, some women of color are also lesbians, or lesbians become motivated due to their community focus as members of the gay and lesbian community and their political ideology (e.g., environmentalism). These "real life" multiple identities of women do not make the types of motivational conditions mutually exclusive.

This discussion raises the question about the merit of creating and discussing three motivational types as though they were distinct separate entities; there are, after all, some women who claim that there is more than one motivational type that brought them to activism. I argue that the creation of three ideal types serves as a distinction between different levels of abstraction.

Diagnosis is the most personal and least abstract motivational type, however, activism only emerges when the personal experience of being diagnosed or misdiagnosed is complemented by political consciousness. The third motivational type, the political-ideological approach, is the counterpiece. This approach to a disease is the motivational type with the highest level of abstraction. Such abstraction, however, materializes as activism only when women's political beliefs or identities are complemented by a personal connection to the disease. This personal connection ranges on a continuum from the most unfortunate circumstance—that is, the woman having the disease herself—to having a person in one's life who is living with the disease.

Hence the ideal types of motivational forces for activism can be distinguished by the different weight of each of the two components—the personal relationship and the political relationship to the disease. This explanation for activism is more complex than the commonly perceived explanations of solidarity and self-interest.

CHAPTER 5

Collective Identity Processes about Sexuality and Gender

While previous chapters connected activism to the various personal identities of participants, the next two chapters focus on collective identities and how they are connected to activism. This first emphasizes how sexual orientation and gender are negotiated in both movements. The second discusses movement strategies for negotiating diversity and building coalitions.

What is meant by collective identity and personal identity? Straight women and lesbians are involved in both movements, a fact that refers to women's personal identities as straight or lesbian women or their social location without indicating how these different sexual identities are shaping the two movements on a collective level. This chapter will do just that—present the collective identities of the two movements with regard to sexual orientation and gender. Although I limit my discussion to the AIDS and breast cancer movements, this discussion has broader implications for other social movements. I argue implicitly that while sexuality and gender are important issues to be negotiated in every social movement, the AIDS and cancer movements present two extremes of this negotiation process. The cancer movement exemplifies one extreme type of movement in that sexual orientation is not an issue of importance in the movement. The AIDS movement exemplifies the opposite and is a movement heavily shaped by issues of sexuality and consequently assists in publicizing the politics of sexuality.

Collective identity

Collective identity is more complex than describing the activists' social locations and different from counting the variety of personal identities of the activists involved. To understand the concept of collective identity, it is helpful to incorporate William Gamson's distinction between the three layers in which collective identity is embedded.[1] The first layer is the specific movement organization (a specific cancer or AIDS organization), the second layer is the movement (AIDS movement or cancer movement), and the third layer is the solidary group (e.g., lesbians, communities of color, and women).

These three layers explain the locus of collective identity and define it as a sociocultural construct and not an individual identity. Collective identity is "manifested through the language and symbols by which it is publicly expressed—in styles of dress, language, demeanor, and discourse."[2] Collective identity, then, is expressed through practices performed on different layers. These practices are consciously chosen after a long discussion within the movement (the second level of identity) or an organization (the first level of identity), or they can be unconscious practices, such as using a language that is derived from an assumed educational background. Nancy Whittier argues that collective identity formation is the outcome of process and is not static:

> In the process of constructing a collective identity, challenging groups adopt labels for themselves (such as "feminist"), draw lines between insiders and outsiders, and develop interpretive frameworks, a political consciousness through which members understand the world. Of course, "collective identities" exist only as far as real people agree upon, enact, argue over, and internalize them; group definitions have no life of their own, and they are constantly changing rather than static.[3]

I have already laid out who the women are and what their differences are in terms of social location when they enter AIDS and breast cancer activism. This chapter focuses on understanding the world and the political consciousness that these various members have achieved, through negotiating and defining AIDS and breast cancer activism on a collective level.

I have consistently referred to AIDS activism as framed around sexism, racism, classism, and sexual orientation, whereas breast cancer activism addresses sexism and the environment. In this chapter I discuss these collective identities and uncover how they maintain a movement's constituency and bring about the eventual success of the movement.

Negotiating gender within cancer activism

Although both movements share a collective identity around gender oppression and sexism, the expression of this identity is different. The cancer movement has organized around a feminist analysis of cancer, arguing that cancer is a political issue that affects women.[4] Here I am concentrating on the specifics of a gender analysis that informs the collective identity at the second level, the movement level.

There are women in the cancer movement who view themselves as feminists as well as women who do not embrace a feminist identity. This creates the situation that the collective feminist identity is negotiated between politically experienced feminists and women with no prior political experience or feminist analysis.[5] For the cancer movement, the outcome of the negotiation process is a feminist collective identity best characterized as liberal or positivist feminism.[6] Liberal or positivist feminism is a type of feminism that seeks to solve gender oppression predominantly through equality. This feminism demands that women have to be represented on all societal levels without necessarily challenging the underlying structures. With regard to cancer, this means, among other things, obtaining equal funding for women's diseases and men's diseases and guaranteeing clinical trials that include women.

This type of liberal feminism frames the cancer movement's approach and actions. Gender is used as a dominant and fixed category, while an analysis of the multiplicity and interconnectedness of gender with other identities such as race, class, and sexual orientation is missing. Whereas the cancer movement puts forward an ideology that claims to be inclusive of *all* women, in reality, the differences among various women, whether black, poor, or lesbian, are not incorporated into the movement's culture. Officially, the cancer movement's agenda is to demand

> improve[d] *access* to high quality breast cancer screening, diagnosis, treatment, and care for all women, particularly the

underserved and uninsured, through legislation and beneficial changes in the regulation and delivery of breast health care. [emphasis in original][7]

Despite displaying an inclusiveness, the movement and individual organizations have created a culture that is white, middle class, and heterosexual. This is different from saying that white heterosexual women are active in the movement, since lesbians, working-class women, and women of color are also part of it. My argument is that the movement culture has been created because of the kind of feminist collective identity prevalent at the second level of cancer activism. A liberal feminist collective identity suggests that we share common ground because we are all women. This liberal approach downplays our differences and their consequences on women's lives, while at the same time it claims to be inclusive of women from all walks of life.

Before I debunk this myth of inclusivity, note that in the debate between *breast cancer* and *cancer* movement those opting for the more "generic" *cancer* do a similar injustice to the notion of inclusivity.[8] The *cancer* organizations claim that their goal is to be inclusive to women with *all* types of cancer, which creates a type of neutrality as though it did not matter what type of cancer women have. I am persuaded by many breast cancer activists who claim that it has a different effect on a woman's identity if she has had a breast removed or if part of her intestines have been removed.

> [W]hen I was a teenager, the two women who raised me both had cancer; one had breast cancer, the other had stomach and intestinal cancer. The one who had breast cancer never recovered. I mean by that, she physically got well, but she never emotionally recovered from the whole process of having her body invaded—first by the disease and then by the medical community because at that time it was all the full radical mastectomy. . . . So this was a real violation. [breast cancer activist]

While women with different types of cancer definitely share commonalities, as much as women share the commonality of gender oppression, the ideology of women with *all* types of cancer suggests a false neutrality between different types of the disease. To deny that the immediate physical realities and the stigma attached to certain types of cancer are different shortchanges women's different experiences.[9]

Although such a vision of inclusivity may be well intentioned, it suggests a false neutrality and equality between the real differences operating in women's lives.

The myth of neutrality and inclusivity

Despite the cancer movement's self-presentation as neutral in regard to sexual orientation, race, and class, I argue that it gives the societal dominant norms a preeminent status. Simply claiming in writing that an organization is open to *all* women, regardless of sexual orientation, class, or race, does not create diversity. On the contrary, this so-called neutrality, or gesture toward inclusivity, creates a culture that operates in the default mode—a mode in which the dominant culture becomes normative. If issues of diversity are not openly addressed, the organizational culture falls back on the dominant norms of larger society, such as being heterosexual, middle class, and white. A culture dominated by societal norms requires that outsiders have to challenge existing structures and fight to be heard. One activist describes how hard it is to bring issues up once the normative culture—in this case, the middle class—is already firmly established.

> There are women in the [organization] who might identify the [organization] as a middle-class group. I mean I feel more strongly about this issue than about the issue of gay and straight because my background is very working class and I have all those sensitivities around being working class. And I cringe when somebody in the group will say, well, we are a middle-class group and I say, wait a minute, you just totally excluded me. I don't say it, I think it. . . . So I get very sensitive and then what happens is I don't speak up and I don't say it because all that class stuff, all these class phenomena come into play, and in addition I sit back and feel angry. And so the next time somebody says that I am gonna confront them on that. And I am gonna say, when you identify this as a middle-class group, you are excluding some of us whose background is not middle class. I am gonna say it. [cancer movement]

While feminists argue that gender neutrality is a myth, cancer activists who consider themselves feminists fail to apply this knowledge to sexuality, race, and class.[10] Therefore, cancer activists are gender-cognizant and created their movement and organizations according to a feminist vision; their gender analysis is based on what sociologist Chrys Ingraham calls "heterogender."[11]

Cancer activism evolved from the women's health movement. It was the women's health movement of the 1970s, and feminists at that time were criticized for their heterogender culture.[12] Despite these earlier criticisms of heterofeminism, the cancer movement nevertheless displays heteroculture.

In chapter 6, I will expand on this by stating that this understanding of gender is also white and middle class.

Negotiating sexuality in cancer versus AIDS activism

The cancer movement's guiding liberal feminism defines sexual orientation narrowly. It is an issue of personal choice that belongs in the private sphere instead of the political one. Accordingly, sexual orientation is unaddressed within this movement. The only exceptions are lesbian cancer organizations or the efforts of individual lesbian activists, who take a different stand.[13]

This is one of the main differences between AIDS and cancer activism. Although women within breast cancer activism become affirmed in their identity as women, such affirmation is narrow. If they are also lesbians, women of color, or poor, cancer activism does not provide them with a similar affirmation of their identities. Within AIDS activism, the complexity or multiplicity of women's lives is acknowledged more fully.

The difference in affirmation of identities in these movements stands for two cultures or the presence of different collective identities. The culture of AIDS activism displays openness and visibility around sexual identities. In other words, the collective identity of the AIDS movement regarding sexual orientation is visible and open, which does not mean gay. In the cancer movement, however, sexual orientation is unaddressed and silenced.

While interviewing AIDS and cancer activists, my questions about sexual identity were well received by women AIDS activists. Among cancer activists, on the other hand, questions about sexual orientation were often perceived as being inappropriate or beside the point of cancer activism. These reactions were independent from respondents' personal sexual identity. Within AIDS activism, straight women and lesbians alike answered questions about sexual orientation in a matter-of-fact way and with eloquence. Many straight and lesbian women within cancer activism framed sexual orientation as an issue that had no bearing on cancer activism, since cancer is not a sexually transmitted disease. This indicates that a woman's sexual orientation is understood as an issue of personal choice rather than as a political issue. Within AIDS activism, on the other hand, lesbians and most straight women were comfortable discussing and presenting the issue of sexual orientation as a political issue and as one aspect of cultural diversity that needed to be incorporated in political activism.

A movement's collective identity is therefore not determined by one's personal social location or personal identity, since straight women and lesbians are found in both movements. But knowledge about sexual orientation and its sociocultural implications is only found within AIDS activism. In addition, the movement's collective identity in regard to sexual orientation is also independent from the actual incidence of disease among straight women and lesbians, since some argue that the likelihood of lesbians developing breast cancer is higher than lesbians' risk of contracting HIV.[14]

The majority of my respondents from the cancer movement argued that sexual orientation should not be highlighted within cancer activism, since the disease itself does not make a distinction between their sexual orientation.[15] One can go further with this argument and add that many diseases occur in men and women, poor and rich, and whites and people of color. Such thinking uses the biomedical conditions of the disease as the model for the world of activism, arguing that since cancer does not discriminate whether you are poor, lesbian, or of color, activism should not distinguish on those terms either. Such thinking renders invisible the differences between women's worlds—whether they are poor, lesbian, or of color. One woman of color speaks about this by referring to cultural differences in regard to cancer:

> I know that Latinos have different needs and that there are cultural ways in which we respond to cancer. Not that the cancer itself is different. But you know the big issue here is women in general. Every community has different needs and every community has different issues. [cancer movement, woman of color]

Further, there is ample evidence in health services research that demographics such as age, socioeconomic status, and race affect patients' treatment and survival. But the cancer movement's liberal feminism tries to dispense with these differences that are so essential to those of us who live as non-whites, non-middle class, or non-heterosexual. One straight woman, for example, called sexual orientation a demographic similar to one's birthplace:

> There is no model of how to be a lesbian or how to be a straight woman in the breast cancer movement. . . . I mean a [medical] researcher might have a reason for finding out sexual orientation so they can develop specific statistics. But why would you want to do it in a political group? . . . [I]t's a demographic you might want to know if you are doing [medical] research, but it wouldn't have any bearing on a political group in my thinking. . . . That's a personal choice. [cancer movement, straight]

Such consciousness about sexual orientation has had the effect of invisibilizing lesbians. When sexual orientation is understood in such personal terms, it is not important that the cancer organizations are designed to cater to *all* women. As Adrienne Rich stated fifteen years ago,

> [A]ny theory or cultural/political creation that treats lesbian existence as a marginal or less "natural" phenomenon, as mere "sexual preference," or as the mirror image of either heterosexual or male homosexual relations is profoundly weakened thereby, whatever its other contributions. Feminist theory can no longer afford merely to voice a toleration of "lesbianism" as an "alternative lifestyle," or make token allusion to lesbians.[16]

Contrary to minimizing sexual orientation to a personal choice, AIDS activism is concerned about sexual orientation as an issue of cultural diversity that needs to be addressed. One straight AIDS activist speaks eloquently about the importance of sexual orientation and exemplifies how sexual orientation is perceived differently between AIDS and cancer activism.

> [I]f we are not doing enough for lesbian persons, I would be the first one to say we need to do something about it. And then I support one of my colleagues to start a group of support for lesbians that are care providers. I think the issue is more supporting each other in the work that we do as women and also supporting the issues that each one of us has. As a

lesbian my colleague will have very different issues than I have. And I think that if we go back again to suffering, I think lesbians suffer a lot more than I do, because I am accepted, you know. I am a heterosexual woman and I do the norm, and I have a son, and I have a husband. But you know, a lesbian has to fight to be happy, has to fight to be able to have a partner, and to be happy with that partner. And they have to fight in their own families to be accepted by their own families, you know what I mean? I think that, because I am a heterosexual woman, I have more doors that are open to me. Then how do I work with my friends who are lesbians or my colleagues? I think it's important to look at it that way. [AIDS movement, straight]

This woman's position on sexual orientation shows that she recognizes the political importance of sexual orientation in a heterosexist society, which is essentially a system of oppression to lesbians. Heterosexism refers to a system of advantages and privileges for heterosexuals that implies the exclusion and oppression of any non-heterosexual behavior and practices, identities, and communities.[17] As a straight woman, she is aware of her privileged position and understands that the issue of sexual orientation involves more than the issue of HIV transmission. Claiming that cancer is not sexually transmitted, however, cancer activists defend their own lack of discussion concerning sexuality. They claim that AIDS activists need to address sexual orientation, since AIDS is a sexually transmitted disease, whereas cancer activists do not need to address it, because cancer is not a sexually transmitted disease.

Culture of AIDS organizations

AIDS activism overtly addresses sexual orientation at all levels of collective identity, whether at the movement level (second level) or at the level of individual organizations (first level). A number of organizations exist that have emerged from and are based in the gay, people of color, or other marginalized communities. Some organizations are characterized by serving a particular type of clientele, such as substance abusers. While all of these organizational types share an openness about sexual orientation, the individual organizational culture differs.

Most gay community-based organizations move beyond mere openness with regard to sexual orientation; instead, they display a gay culture. By gay culture, I mean an environment in which the societal counterculture of being gay and lesbian is normative.[18] The culture of organizations other than gay community based is more determined by other factors, such as a collective racial identity or norms of the respective communities that are targeted for education and prevention (e.g., substance abusers). These organizations' culture, which is open about sexual orientation, can be referred to as "gay positive." "Gay positive" refers to an environment that has not one normative sexual orientation, but being gay or lesbian is openly addressed and treated as equal to being heterosexual or any other sexual orientation.[19]

Lesbians who are involved in gay community organizations express a high level of satisfaction about the ways in which their sexual orientation is embraced on this level of AIDS activism. These lesbians describe their activism within gay community organizations as a positive experience, because the support of their lesbian identity is unique and runs counter to their daily life experiences. One activist voices her experience within a gay community-based organization in the following way:

> It's an incredible place to be a lesbian in. You don't check any part of yourself at the door. In fact, you are encouraged to be more outrageous than you might be, which is certainly a different experience than being at another work place. I feel saddened of the idea that at some point I won't be here and I'll be back in some regular world job. . . . I think, people love the people here and love mostly that it's kind of, a place, an environment in terms of community. So, that's been really great. [AIDS movement, lesbian]

The sense of community and the connection to which this activist refers is based on the commonality of being supported as "gay or lesbian." This is a unique experience and is different from being "out" in an open-minded environment that is gay supportive or "gay positive."

Given that being gay or lesbian is the norm within gay community-based organizations, straight women are very conscious about being outsiders. While women of color have ample life experiences that run counter to societal norms, it could be that straight white women will have more of a problem with their alien status in a gay-dominated environment. Straight white women can merely draw upon their limited experience of gender oppression, which is counterbalanced by white skin privilege. One straight white activist who used to be involved in AIDS activism and then moved on to cancer activism compares her experiences of being straight in an AIDS environment to a cancer environment.

> [Within AIDS activism,] there was definitely a feeling of in and out based on what your sexual orientation was. Not if you are a woman or a man, because you were in or out based on whether you were straight or gay. . . . I wrote about what it was like to be a sexual minority, to be a heterosexual sexual minority in a predominantly gay area. That's a fascinating experience. In terms of the breast cancer group, I mean I know who is gay, I have a pretty good antenna for it because I hung out with gay people for a long time. I can figure who is gay very easily. It's something that you know, you don't have to be in your face about it, it's something that becomes obvious once you talk to somebody. . . . [Within cancer activism] it doesn't really matter whether you are gay or straight. [formerly within the AIDS movement, later the cancer movement]

While this activist's straight sexual identity was against the norm within a gay community-based AIDS organization, she felt more comfortable, however, within the cancer movement. Within the cancer movement, lesbians are not "in someone's face about sexual orientation," since lesbians appeared to mostly "check that part of themselves at the door" before they entered cancer organizations. This illustrates the point that, despite the cancer movement's denial that it was making one sexual orientation more important than the other, it operates in a straight culture.

Lesbian identity and cancer activism

The majority of lesbian cancer activists describe the culture of the cancer movement as neutral, or they regard it as tolerant and accepting of lesbians. Although the atmosphere may appear superficially neutral and tolerant toward lesbians, feminist thinker Elizabeth Spelman states this about tolerance:

> "Yes, I'll tolerate you" leaves me the same. If one is in a position to allow someone else to do something, one is also in a position to keep that person from doing it. To tolerate your speaking is to refrain from exercising the power I have

to keep you from speaking. In tolerating you I have done nothing to change the fact that I have more power and authority than you do. And of course I don't have to listen to what you say.[20]

If the atmosphere toward lesbians is merely tolerant, then lesbians are invisibilized.

Lesbians are mostly invisibilized within cancer activism, because sexual orientation is not openly addressed. Such silence around sexual orientation may create an atmosphere of tolerance toward lesbians, but the milieu is nonetheless heterosexist. I argue that cancer activism takes place in heterosexist conditions, which does not imply the existence of homophobia, which generally does not pervade cancer activism. Here I argue that while heterosexism and homophobia are overlapping concepts, I understand homophobia to mean irrational fear of homosexuality and hatred of homosexuals, which might lead to acts of discrimination or violence in their most extreme form. On the contrary, heterosexism refers to the taken-for-granted norm of heterosexuality, the systematic privileging of heterosexual behavior and identity.[21] Hence, the cancer activists' atmosphere of tolerance is created through a lack of statements about sexual orientation. Such tolerance is characterized by an absence of voiced homophobia, but the overall silence about sexual orientation is still heterosexist. In that sense, the difference between heterosexism and homophobia is gradual. Whereas heterosexism is more pervasive, homophobia is a possible second step in a heterosexist or heterogender culture. Overall, my claim is that cancer activism's culture is heterosexist without being homophobic: it is nonsupportive of lesbians' sexual identity, and lesbians are merely acknowledged or supported in their gender identity. My position on the cancer movement's culture is, however, not shared by the majority of lesbian cancer activists whom I interviewed.

> [We] never really [talk] much about the fact that we are a mixed group of lesbians and straight women. It was just sort of taken for granted and I don't think anyone thinks of this. But it hasn't much to do with what we are doing.
> *Interviewer:* So how do you find out then about each other, who are the lesbians and who are the straight women?
> How do I know that there is roughly 50 percent? Once someone starts to mention a partner or something. It's like the whole matrix of community. I find out that [member] knows

> my friend from way back and they know each other from [a
> lesbian group]. [Another lesbian who is a member of the group]
> is a good friend of friends of mine in [some location]. You
> know, you begin to find out. And in fact there are some people
> I am not even sure whether or not they are lesbians. So there
> is the group that I know, the group that I am not sure of and
> a group that I am pretty sure are straight. And yet most people
> until you have a sort of hazard conversation or just happen to
> have the chance to talk about something personal, you just
> don't necessarily know. [cancer movement, lesbian]

This activist, who finds out through the "grapevine" who is a lesbian
and who is uncertain about some members' sexual orientation, speaks
to the invisibilizing of lesbians within cancer organizations. I argue
that this is the opposite to what feminist culture used to express with
the slogan, "The personal is political." Within cancer activism, feminist culture is characterized by an absence of politicizing from social
locations. Instead, the culture is much more dominated by a detached,
scientific, and therefore depersonalized atmosphere that stems from
the cancer movement's goal to focus on prevention by focusing on the
environment.

Some lesbian cancer activists are more critical of the heterocultural
atmosphere within cancer activism. Lesbian cancer organizations, for
instance, are aware that they are the only organizations to raise the
issue of sexuality consistently. If not for these specific lesbian organizations, the movement would only speak from its heterogender
analysis. Other lesbians suggest that making sexual orientation a
nonissue might be a strategy to maintain the peace. Further, some of
these lesbians argue that as long as no overt homophobic comments
or instances occur, the movement might be better off ignoring the
issue.

This points more to the fact that the relationship between lesbians
and straight women in the cancer movement is uneasy at best. This
has been acknowledged by some lesbians and straight women in the
privacy of the interview situation. Despite the lesbian respondents'
portrayal of the cultural atmosphere as non-homophobic, they talked
also about experiences with straight women that revealed their lack of
language when talking with lesbians or their lack of knowledge about
lesbian lives. One lesbian activist pointed out that some of the straight
women might have never consciously met a lesbian before working
with them on the issue of breast cancer.

I sat at a fund-raising dinner . . . [and this straight] woman with breast cancer, middle class, upper middle class, suburban . . . was sitting next to me at the table. I knew her . . . she knew I was a lesbian and I was there with [my partner] and she had a couple of drinks [and] we were all waiting for dinner and she leans over to me and said, "Can I ask you some questions?" And I said, "You can ask me anything you want" And she said, "I know you are a lesbian." "That's right," I said. "But you have kids?" And I said, "Yeah, because I was married right out of college." And she was, I mean, she was totally blown away. So she had never talked to anyone who has identified themselves as a lesbian before. So she took this opportunity to kind of educate herself. So I answered her questions and those kinds of things . . . that's part of, I think, what the breast cancer movement is, I don't want to say struggling with, because I think those of us who are lesbians who are involved in this work feel that it's so important that we are not wasting a lot of time with other women, with straight women's issues. We [are] not gonna stop the movement and say, "Time out here. We want to make sure that none of you are homophobic." Because women are dying, 46,000 women a year are dying. I don't care what their sexual orientation is. I mean they are dying. And we don't have time to deal with this. I mean we deal on a personal kind of level when it comes up. But I don't think there is a strategic kind of decision that was made to minimize it. [cancer movement, lesbian]

Consequently, most lesbian activists have decided to address homophobia, either on a personal level or when it emerges within the context of cancer activism. But the prevailing heterosexism goes mostly unchallenged. While the convictions of lesbians are not to rock the boat and to limit confrontations to overt homophobia, they expressed excitement and hope about the new ways of bonding with straight women. One activist said, "I just haven't been involved in groups where I had contact with straight white suburban housewives" [cancer movement]. Overall, the lesbians believe that cancer activism is an educational opportunity for straight women in sexual diversity. The lesbians hope that straight women's exposure to lesbians will dissolve any concealed homophobia among straight women, with hopes that the ground will eventually be prepared for a culture free of heterosexism.

Given that differences around sexual orientation are not openly addressed within cancer activism, straight women also have an unspoken stand on the issue. The majority of straight women expressed how comfortable they feel, since the movement welcomes all women, regardless of their sexual orientation and other identities.

Some straight respondents express gratitude to the lesbians who started the cancer movement. They suspect that, without these lesbians, there might not be a cancer movement today.

> I think the lesbian community has been very instrumental in getting women from this subservient attitude out into the open. I mean they have laid a lot of ground work for many women's issues. . . . I don't know when that would have happened otherwise, if it was just all happy heterosexual housewives . . . it probably might not have happened. . . . We really should be very grateful to the lesbian community for that because I really think they have been very instrumental. [cancer movement, straight]

A few straight women reflect on the uneasiness between straight women and lesbians.[22] In private conversations, in an all-straight environment, discomfort is at times expressed about lesbianism. This discomfort is expressed by straight women inside of the movement as well as by straight women outside of the movement who keep a distance from a group that is mixed with regard to sexuality. One straight woman talks about the tension that the "lesbian issue" causes straight women outside of the movement.

> I see that other people have a little bit of a problem [with the lesbian issue]. . . . Periodically there is a little bit of stress. A number of my [straight] friends [who are non-members] . . . come to the rally and see a lot of lesbians. Last year, two lesbian women spoke, one of them who had undergone a bone marrow transplant. They talked about what it was like for them as a couple or family. A number of my friends from out here said, "I wish you had told me that that's gonna happen because that's something I wouldn't felt so comfortable bringing my kids." I was disgusted and outraged [cancer movement, straight]

The straight cancer activist was outraged about the homophobic reaction of her friend, who is not a movement member.

But nevertheless, within the movement, the issue of lesbian visibility creates an unacknowledged friction.

> There may be some uncomfortableness with that distinction [lesbians and straight women]. . . . I mean there are people [inside of the movement] who would like to see the leadership change and become a straight leadership rather than a lesbian leadership.
> *Interviewer:* Why is that?
> I just think they would like to see their own personal agenda pushed. They feel like we are concentrating more on the lesbian community. I don't see it that way. . . . [Some straight women] just feel that it's time for a difference [in leadership]. . . . For the most part, I think [lesbians and heterosexuals] get along fine. But there is always a power struggle and you know, we have elections coming up so that's why I am very cognizant of this right now. So people [some straight women within the movement] like to see a change. [cancer movement, straight]

This kind of information that has been shared by lesbian and straight cancer activists proves how uneasy the relationship is between lesbians and straight women. The cancer movement's resistance to openly deal with sexual orientation may work against the movement's future long-term success, although it worked in the short term. Movement strategies such as balancing short-term solutions and long-term success with regard to diversity are discussed in chapter 6.

A different strategy of dealing with sexual orientation has been chosen by at least one other organization.

> I think it was the right decision for LCCP [Lesbian Community Cancer Project] to organize with the word "lesbian" in it, because it was decided from the beginning that that was the primary group of people it wanted to do outreach to, and that the founding members by and large were coming out of the lesbian community. And they really wanted that to be right up front in their identity. So that even though it was also inclusive, it would guarantee that women who were outside of the lesbian community would have to have lesbian positive attitudes to join, whereas to say we are women rather than lesbian and you can say it is inclusive, but it turns it around. [cancer movement]

The LCCP's approach to inclusivity follows one strain of lesbian feminist theory. Lesbian theorist Bette Tallen argues in favor of using "lesbian" as the inclusive term that also applies to non-lesbians, whereas "women" is not inclusive.

> Usually when lesbians write theory they mean to be inclusive of any woman who is willing to identify with a lesbian context. Perhaps it is time that non-lesbians cease to see lesbian as an exclusionary term that does not include them. Lesbian may well be far more inclusive than either feminist or woman, as non-lesbians use those terms.[23]

The vast majority of cancer organizations that have been started by a majority of lesbians, however, take the opposite approach. This approach assumes that any group of lesbians is called a group of women as soon as a single straight woman is among them.[24] This strategy among feminist cancer activists on the one hand and a male-dominated AIDS movement culture on the other hand leads to lesbian invisibility. Lesbian theorist Julia Penelope claims:

> Our invisibility, even to ourselves, is at least partially due to the fact that our identity is subsumed by two groups: women and gays. As a result, Lesbian issues seem to find their way, by neglect or elimination, to the bottom of both liberation agendas. The liberation of Lesbians is supposed to wait for the liberation of all women, or be absorbed and evaporate into the agenda compiled by gay men. Instead of creating free space for ourselves, we allow men to oppress us invisibly in both categories, as "women" or as "gays," without even the token dignity of being named "Lesbians." How we name ourselves determines how visible we are, even to each other.[25]

Gay male AIDS culture

While I previously discussed that sexual orientation is openly addressed within AIDS activism, I also want to acknowledge how gender is negotiated in the movement. Because AIDS is framed as a gay male disease, and because AIDS organizations were formed mostly by gay men, the culture of AIDS activism started from a gay male perspective. The support that lesbians experience regarding their sexual identity is due to an openness that gay men created. This means that within neither the cancer nor the AIDS movement did lesbians create a culture of their own. To recapitulate Penelope, lesbian issues slide to the bottom of both movements' agendas. Within the cancer movement, lesbians participate in a heterosexual culture as argued earlier, whereas lesbians in the AIDS movement excel with regard to their sexual identity in the space that gay men have created. The space within the AIDS movement is gay space, which has to be read as gay male space and is therefore different from having a lesbian culture.[26]

Many lesbians embrace and appreciate gay male culture for its comfort regarding sexuality. One lesbian activist reminisces about the time before AIDS activism, claiming, "Lesbians learned about sex from gay men, because lesbians couldn't talk about and think [about] sex to save their lives. They were just sort of on a totally other path" [AIDS movement].

The sexually affirmative culture of AIDS activism is in opposition to some segments of the women's movement today and was even more so during the "sex wars"[27] that raged in the women's movement around the time AIDS activism began.

> I was a part of the really bitter fights within the women's movement around sexuality and pornography and the kind of definition of sexuality. . . . When the battles got really brutal in the women's movement and in the lesbian movement about sex, I think I made a decision to do AIDS work because it was a place where the politics that I had around sexuality were welcome. You needed to be able to talk about sex and you needed to be able to talk about class and race and you needed to be able to talk about sexual orientation and all of those things were really necessary components of doing AIDS work, especially early on in the epidemic. So I think a lot was in reaction to the battles in the women's movement over sexuality. I just thought I am out of here, you know. I don't want to be in a movement that is so limited in the way it understands desire and I am gonna go to a place where I actually [will] be able to use my gift as an organizer. [AIDS movement]

These activists appreciated the gay male culture for its appreciation of sexuality, and some of the HIV-positive women welcomed the vigor with which gay men politicized AIDS and fought for funding for AIDS research. One straight, HIV-positive AIDS activist summed this up by saying, "If it wasn't for gay men, I probably would be dead by now" [AIDS movement].

Next to these positive aspects of the gay male culture, straight and lesbian women AIDS activists point to its downside, which is the sexism and misogyny of men. One straight activist talks about her struggle in male-dominated AIDS organizations.

> Unfortunately in most of these places, there are men there [in AIDS organizations] that want their money and they are the ones that decide. . . . [W]hat I see is that most of the companies [her term for AIDS organizations] are run by men and the women have no chance to say what they want. . . . It's all about power, you know. The man is here [gestures up] and the woman is here [gestures lower]. You are there [in an AIDS organization] because they have to have you there as a woman, to say that they have women. But who makes the decision there [in an AIDS organization] are the men, it won't be the women. [AIDS movement]

Despite the efforts of women activists who confronted the sexism of male AIDS activists, sexism by men in the movement is still pervasive, as the following statement by a lesbian AIDS activist indicates:

> It's a pretty sexist place. . . . [The men] don't get women's issues. And the senior management team is four women and four men. Four lesbians and four gay men. And it is as if it was run by eight men. You know, we are just outnumbered. I mean there are four of us and four of them and we just, you cannot raise issues of sexism. They don't get it. They sort of have this feeling, oh they have to deal with homophobia so why should they have to deal with issues of sexism. [AIDS movement, lesbian]

Women activists, with and without HIV/AIDS, white and of color, and lesbian and straight, all describe similar experiences with male activists. These negative experiences of AIDS activism within a male culture stand in contrast to the positive aspects of a pro-sex gay culture and a vigorous fight for the funding of AIDS services and research.

This indicates a pattern within the AIDS movement that is different than the cancer movement's. Women AIDS activists who admit that there has been much improvement over the years still bemoan sexism by some male activists that can permeate AIDS activism. This challenges my previous claim about AIDS activism that targets sexism. My claim stems from the fact that my research focus is on women AIDS activists who have put sexism on the agenda of the AIDS movement. Moreover, I also defend the AIDS movement in general, because, collectively, it stands for the fight against sexism. Women's accounts of sexist men refer to the leadership of some AIDS organizations, but the movement's collective identity entails fighting sexism. This distinction will become clearer in chapter 6, in which I distinguish collective identity further by identity practices.

In summary

Within this chapter, sexuality and gender have been presented according to their different levels of importance within both movements. These movements have both lesbian and straight activists, but sexual orientation is a prominent political issue within AIDS activism. In cancer activism, however, sexual orientation is invisibilized. Many women within the cancer movement argue that a working relationship between lesbians and straight women is an accomplishment. Instead, I argue that this working relationship takes place under heterosexual rules and in a heterosexist environment that has been created by straight women due to their lack of awareness of their privileged position.

While this discussion of sexuality and gender was limited to these two health-related movements, these issues are also applicable to other movements. Lesbian and straight women either participate already in many more than the two movements discussed here, or they should be sought out as participants for other movements. While contemporary social movements commonly pay attention to the issue of gender, any social movement that is truly concerned about achieving a broad base through cultural diversity also has to pay attention to the politics of sexual orientation.

The reality is that the cancer movement's culture concerning sexual orientation is the standard for many social movements, whereas the AIDS movement's sexuality politics is the exception. To support this argument, I like to quote from the experiences of "Resist," a group that funds organizations working for social change through grants. Resist requests that organizations applying for funding answer a battery of questions. Among them is a question about the diversity of the group in regard to age, race, sexual orientation, class, and gender, and there is a question about incentives that the applicant offers to increase diversity.[28] While most of the organizations are capable of giving good descriptions of their class, racial, sex, and age makeup, the request for information about members' sexual orientation, however, causes difficulty for some applicants. On behalf of "Resist," Larry Goldsmith summarizes the organizations' responses regarding sexual orientation:

> Some groups profess not to know, or else not to care, or they tell us they would not presume to ask, or that they think it inappropriate to pry—but they usually assure us, in any case, that they do not discriminate. Consider the following examples: One group notes that "age ranges from 20 to 50. Racial characteristics are predominantly Caucasian, though among these seven are Brazilian and one is Puerto Rican. One of our core members is African American. Another is commonly perceived in the U.S. as indigenous, although in Brazil she would merely be considered 'mulatta.' "
>
> Along with this detailed description of racial composition, they also state that the group is 60 percent women, and, by way of addressing class and income level, they provide a list of members' occupations. This same group, however, that can describe so precisely the race, sex, and occupational profile of its membership, also notes that they "have no information on the sexual orientation of our members and regard it as inappropriate to solicit such information."[29]

This shows that the cancer movement's culture is more or less normative among other social change movements. In chapter 6, cultural diversity within movements will be discussed in the context of collective identity, along with the related issues of movement strategies and coalition building.

CHAPTER 6

Diversity and Movement Strategies

Thus far, most of the discussion on collective identity negotiating processes has focused on sexuality and gender and on the ways in which these two issues are dealt with on the organizational and the movement levels. The third level in which collective identity is embedded, solidary (e.g., women, African Americans, and workers), will come more into play when strategies and coalition building are discussed.

Another useful tool for understanding and evaluating the collective identities of the breast cancer and the AIDS movements is Sharon Kurtz's concept of identity practices.[1] According to Kurtz, identity practices are movements' social practices that have a cumulative effect; taken together, they shape the collective identity of a movement. She argues that "[A]t each level, a collective identity involves an ideological position which offers an analysis of the problem the movement faces, implying solutions and potential allies,"[2] and that these practices are generally not the outcome of direct and conscious decision making by organizations or movements. Kurtz then moves on to list six identity practices: (1) issue/program formulation; (2) framing of the issues and movement; (3) outside support resources drawn in; (4) movement culture; (5) organizational structure; and (6) leadership/ organizational power. Kurtz's listing of identity practices gives social

119

movement researchers tools that allow for an evaluation of movements' collective identities.

Such evaluation of movements' collective identity could be further enhanced by adding a seventh identity practice to Kurtz's list. I suggest adding a seventh identity practice: the distribution or the spending of resources. Any movement makes decisions on spending resources (e.g., time, energy, money). By paying close attention to how the movement distributes resources, another social practice becomes evident. For instance, a movement or an organization might have collected money for the printing and distribution of certain materials. There is, however, not enough money to print all of the materials. Under the conditions of a tight budget, which materials get printed reveals an important identity practice. Does the organization or movement decide to print fewer materials in general but does so in two or more languages? Or will the organization decide to publish more in one language? Furthermore, similar conflicts also occur with regard to time. Maybe a hot line needs to be staffed or room for a support group provided. Most of the time movements or organizations operate under time and money constraints and are forced to choose between different options. Movements' collective identity shows in the choices they make and in their distribution of resources.

For activists, the operationalization of collective identity into identity practices is an important tool as well. Activists' awareness about identity practices gives them tools for intervention. Once an awareness exists about certain social practices that interfere with the movement's pursuit of a politics of diversity, activists can change any practice that is debilitating to the movement's goals.

To illustrate Kurtz's concept of identity practices, I refer once more to the issues of gender and sexuality, discussed in the previous chapter. Her concept of identity practices allows one to specify that AIDS activism consistently invokes the politics of sexuality in all six of Kurtz's identity practices. On the other hand, the cancer movement expresses the politics of sexuality merely within the context of outside support and resources. The issue of gender permeates all identity practices of the cancer movement. On the contrary, the AIDS movement invokes gender in most identity practices but shows definite weaknesses with regard to leadership or organizational power. I will continue to discuss collective identity and cultural diversity by drawing upon issues other than sexuality and gender and by showing how identity practices are shaped by these issues in the two movements.[3]

As noted earlier, the cancer movement's culture has been characterized as liberal feminist. Liberal feminism's approach to diversity is to chop

> women up metaphysically into parts: the part of me in virtue of which I have a particular gender identity, the part of me in virtue of which I am of a particular race, and so on—as if a person's identity were like a patchwork quilt, made up of separable pieces, each with an identity, a history, and a meaning all its own.[4]

Liberal feminist activism around cancer does just that: it highlights that the focus is on *all women* and thereby operates with an additive oppression analysis.[5] The focus is on *all women* because it is assumed that women share a "generic womanness" and that as women *"we"* face a common oppression—gender oppression. As with the differences around sexuality, the universalism about gender oppression represented by the pronoun *"we"* that is prevalent in such liberal feminist thinking takes heterosexual women's experiences, generalizes from these experiences, and treats them as though they are applicable to all women. This practice treats lesbian women as though *"they"* share a womanness with heterosexual women and then, somewhere in their lives, *"they"*—the lesbians—have to deal with something additional— their sexual identity. This liberal feminist perspective on diversity frames not only lesbians but also women of color or poor women as being slightly different from the *"we,"* and requiring something in addition to the generic experience of white heterosexual middle-class women who are at the center of the universal *"we."*[6]

While neither sexual identity is discussed openly nor the politics of sexuality are intended as a movement goal, cancer movement participants do claim that they desire cultural diversity in regard to race and socioeconomic status. For instance, cancer activists readily admit that they are too homogenous in race and class and that so far the movement has failed to attract poor women and women of color as constituencies. This awareness has led to various attempts at overcoming the existing ethnocentrism. One such effort is to name race and class as issues of importance to cancer activism.[7] While this speaks to a certain class and race awareness, it must not be construed as a collective identity that reflects anti-racism and anti-classism. Such a collective identity is nonexistent within the cancer movement. Instead, race and class are generally limited to being addressed only symboli-cally. Race and class within the cancer movement are mostly limited to the identity practice of issue/program formulation.[8] This is consis-tent with this book's contentions in that the cancer movement has no collective identity of anti-racism and anti-classism. One can expect that the movement will not invoke or integrate race and class concerns in all of the movement's identity practices.

Another attempt by the cancer movement was to achieve diversity by building outreach committees. These committees had the goal of recruiting women of color as members. From the feminist thinker Spelman we learn that such attempts to reach out by "adding on" race and class reinforce the existing privilege of white heterosexual middle-class women.[9] As Barbara Omolade has said, "Black women are not white women with color."[10]

The determination that the cancer movement's collective identity lacks culturally diverse practices leads one to ask what culturally di-verse identity practices are. Or what does a collective identity of anti-racism and anti-classism look like? And what does it mean to openly discuss differences around sexuality, race, and class? Posing these questions leads us to strategies for creating diversity by negotiating multiple identities within a movement.

Assessing differences

In order to move toward the goal of collective identities that incor-porate anti-racism and anti-classism in cancer organizing, we need to assess which differences exist between communities of color and white women. Generally it can be stated that cancer activism is now shaped from the racial perspective of whiteness and a middle-class background. This means that concerns of non-white communities and poor women are mostly excluded. I have already given examples[11] that confirm this statement, and now I would like to exemplify this point by focusing on the racially segregated position on mammography. In 1993, mam-mography for women under age fifty caused a controversy, because it appeared that there was no statistically significant reduction in mor-tality for women with breast cancer in this age group. The mammog-raphy controversy sparked a discussion about screening guidelines among public health professionals and cancer activists. While mam-mography proved effective in reducing mortality from breast cancer in women between ages fifty and sixty-nine, its merit in saving the lives of younger and older women is questionable.[12] Some cancer activists have argued that mammography is the cancer establishment's shotgun approach to breast cancer, and that the establishment uses it to make women feel safe and to cover up the fact that nothing is currently available to prevent breast cancer. Other arguments highlight the fact that mammography requires a low dosage of radioactivity. A woman who gets regular mammograms from an early age on might actually have an increased risk of breast cancer due to her cumulative exposure to radiation.[13] The topic of mammography tends to be divisive among cancer activists in general and among my respondents along racial lines. White women tend to take a negative stand on mammography. Cancer activists of color favor free mammography screening and screenings for younger women who have a higher incidence of breast cancer in their communities. Many women of color believe that mammography screening at age fifty is too late for women of color. Women of color testified before the President's Cancer Panel in favor of mammography. They demanded more accessible and timely screening for women in marginalized communities.[14] This shows that a culturally diverse cancer activism would have to be shaped differently. It would have to reframe the movement's stand regarding mammography so that non-white and poor women's perspectives were visible and part of the demands. A possible reframing of the mammography that incorporates women of color's concerns could stress that institutions such as the National Cancer Institute or the American Cancer Society, which make broad statements such as "Women in their forties or older should get screening mammograms on a regular basis," have to be race specific in their recommendations, and to do so they have to evaluate the findings of randomized clinical trials that included women of various races and ethnicities.[15]

Organizing styles

Women of color define feminism differently than white women. Therefore, feminist activism regarding cancer would take on a different style if women of color's perspective became a part of cancer activism's feminist movement culture. One woman of color describes her encounter with the limitation of white feminism:

> [T]he bottom line I got from that was that either you do it one way, you approach breast cancer one way or you don't join. . . . [W]e were talking about fund-raising. And they were talking about having a boat ride to raise money for breast

cancer. I said, "Cool that's fine. But in my community, meaning African-American women and Latina women, people are
really into African clothing and the big thing now is having an
African fashion show. Why don't we have an African fashion
show and feature women with breast cancer to let people see
that I have breast cancer, I am still beautiful, blah blah blah."
Well, even the women in the so-called diversity outreach committee, many of them were against it. And I said, "Why are
you against it?" And they are like, "You know, women are
showing their bodies to men and women are being exploited
blah blah blah." I understand the whole feminist view but in
this particular community that we are dealing with, if we are
modeling clothes for us, to ourselves and not modeling it in
front of men, we don't see that as female gender exploitation.
We see that as celebrating our beauty and this is another example of how we should be able to fight breast cancer in
different ways. Well, the African fashion show did not fly
because the policy was we do not do fashion shows, because
they exploit women. You know [she laughs], I can see if we
were strip teasing or something but it wasn't like that. So we
still have to deal with the difference of philosophies and strategies as to fighting breast cancer. And people have to recognize that there are some barriers that other groups of women
have that they might not have, like the race issue or the socioeconomic issue which they kind of heard about. [cancer movement, woman of color]

From this example, we learn how a multicultural activism would be
different in regard to movement culture. A multicultural activism would
have to choose a feminist movement culture that reflects and integrates the differences in values and practices that exist between the
feminism of women of color and the feminism of white women.

To illustrate some possible solutions to the complicated task of
implementing multicultural identity practices, I rely on the AIDS movement. Contrary to the cancer movement, the AIDS movement's collective identity entails anti-racism and anti-classism. Hence, we should
expect to find identity practices that express the politics of race and
class and multiculturalism in Kurtz's identity practices. It has to be
noted that the AIDS movement did not start as a multicultural movement or with a multicultural collective identity. Instead it expanded its
collective identity to incorporate anti-racism and anti-classism.

For instance, one woman of color who works within the Latina community addressed obstacles that had previously prevented AIDS activists to reach multiple communities. But various cultural conditions were taken into account, and activities have been reorganized appropriately.

> [T]he place, like in the Spanish community, the people are used to being in houses because that's their culture. We don't have so many offices. Like in here [the U.S.], there happens a lot in offices. We are not used to that, culturally we are not. You call somebody to your home that's different, you know. It's like right now, we talk about it and they are willing to come here or another house where they can be helped. But a house, not a [office] building, you know. [AIDS movement, woman of color]

Responding to the differences in conditions that exist, as in this case of the Latina community, shows how the AIDS movement has modified its culture and organizational structure.

The AIDS movement is older, and its collective identity has overcome the nonvisibility of anti-racism and anti-classism. In that it is now an acclaimed part of the AIDS movement's collective identity, it is clear that diversity in identity practices is attainable. Identity practices are subject to change, and such change expresses a movement's awareness to aligning the movement's identity practices with its collective identity. In fact, today's AIDS movement has a different style of activism compared to its beginning years. The movement has worked on modifying identity practices that had been working against multicultural diversity.

One example that shows a gradual implementation of multicultural concerns is HIV prevention work. Today, prevention work through HIV education in communities of color is frequently done by women activists of color. These women have advice for breast cancer activists on how to modify organizing styles so women of color and poor women become engaged.

> Well, the kind of people who do activist stuff tend to be white middle-class people.... But in order to engage African-American and other women of color in things like the breast cancer movement, it has to be approached differently. The [current white, middle-class] structures are formidable for a

lot of people, go to a meeting, raise your hand, and you have Robert's Rules of Order and all that kind of stuff. And for a lot of [non-white] people that's not how they approach illness. Illness is a personal thing. What we were doing about our program, we went out to women, sat down and talked to them in their homes. That's in my experience how you get poor people of color involved in movements. It doesn't mean that they don't go to rallies and stuff like that. But they are not gonna start that way. It had to start with a personal, an inter-personal experience, and then you bring people out. It has to be done in a different way. Middle-class, white women don't tend to engage minority women that way. They don't get in-volved. They only get involved in interpersonal relationships with you on their [white, middle-class] turf. But they don't get involved in interpersonal relationships with women of color on the turf of the women of color. That's not how they oper-ate. This is not a criticism. It's just a description. We live in different worlds . . . people of color, particularly poor people of color, their position is . . . how do I know I can trust you? How do I know that you just don't want to have power over me and tell me what to do? So you have to demonstrate your trustwor-thiness. If they want to engage us, although I am not poor, that's my background, they gonna have to do it differently. [AIDS movement, woman of color]

This activist offered an important lesson to breast cancer activists by naming practices that are rooted in white middle-class activism. As long as breast cancer activism operates in this way, it will not be inviting to and capable of attracting poor women and women of color into the movement. The AIDS activist who spoke so eloquently about movement practices went even further and explained what a cultur-ally sensitive organizing style looked like in the everyday world of AIDS organizing.

Let me tell you how we do things. We are funded to do HIV education in Latina communities. The way we do that and we didn't create it, but the way we do that is that we do some-thing like Tupperware parties. We go to the home of a Latina woman. We make arrangements with them, they invite their friends and relatives and we go and do the education in their homes. They are not gonna come here [office buildings that house AIDS organization] as a group. It's sort of an embarrassment and other kinds of things and there are taboos around that. But they want to know and they have a lot of concerns. But it's done on their turf with their friends and their relatives and their way. That's how we do it. They never come to this agency. . . . It's their home and they are in charge. We underestimate people's desire to have some control over, a sense of control over their own lives. And when people come here we are in control. When they misbehave, we can just put them out. When you go to somebody's home, they are in charge, they are in control and you have to do things the way they want it done, which is all right with me. [AIDS movement, woman of color]

While this account seems anecdotal, it does touch on some important cultural values that bring about different styles of activism.

Choosing strategies

Issues are framed and presented differently in multicultural movements that incorporate collective identities of anti-racism and anti-classism than in movements that are lacking these components. Messages of multicultural movements need to respond to societal conditions of racism and classism. Within AIDS activism, this approach can be found within AIDS prevention messages. For instance, to be effective, AIDS prevention through education has to be broadly defined so the particular aspects of women's lives and identities are reflected. One AIDS activist speaks to this in the following way:

It does seem to me that activism ought to be focused on people's own needs, to be empowered to solve their own problems. . . . So for instance, at this point we don't have any real good answers on how to prevent HIV, we have this like mechanical answer, use a condom or use clean needles. But we don't have the social conditions that would underlie its prevention. We don't have women who can say to their partners use a condom. We don't have social relations between women and men that make that possible. . . . You know, the big challenge right now is for us to examine those social relations and those conditions that are underlying why AIDS is happening at all. AIDS shouldn't be happening anymore. . . .

> And so I think the next 10 years women have to really scramble to come up with a political response. And I think inevitably we will have to make alliances. . . . Here is our poster campaign that tries to talk about the other issues in women's lives besides just tell him to use a condom . . . because these are the things on women's minds: how to raise their children, how to pay the rent. There is one that addresses battering. So I think we're gonna have to build relationships with battered women's groups, with people doing work with substance abuse and women. And really try to form a response that's got all the pieces in it. Instead of just be an AIDS activist or be an AIDS educator. [AIDS movement]

Such broadness in goals and messages is required when the needs of diverse communities are taken into consideration. Messages must speak to real-life situations of diverse populations and not just sum up the bare "mechanics of the issue." While within the breast cancer movement the message of pushing for research that links the causes of cancer to the environment appears to be broad, the movement neglects the smaller steps with which people struggle in their everyday lives. Most women of color argue that the needs of their communities are not addressed by present grassroots cancer organizations, since the current framing of issues neglects to take their needs into consideration. One activist of color argues for the importance of addressing other aspects, such as economic conditions, which dominate life in her community, as opposed to the environmental connection to cancer:

> Needs of survival, simple basic needs, a place to stay, taking care of your family. And the fact that you are, I think that that [the environment] would be a hard sell to this community, especially when you have a community that is sort of segregated right here in the inner city. I mean when we start moving out, number one, you have got to have a job and you got to be making pretty good income and be able to survive once you move out. For instance, . . . [where] one of the major [housing] projects is, they have a rubbish disposal plant right next to this [housing] project. This is where poor people live, you know and so, how are you gonna move all of these families away from this sewage disposal plant, you know? How can you talk to them about environmental control without offering them a means of doing that? I think that the needs of the

> Afro-American community and I don't dispute the fact that there is a need to look at the environment . . . [but] how are we gonna expect people to deal with that realistically? [cancer movement, woman of color]

These different conditions are frequently reflected in various identity practices. Social events such as conferences or the cancer movement's discourse reflect the concerns of white middle-class communities. In communities of color, discussions center instead on health insurance and access to treatment. Among white cancer activists, the discourse is a scientific one about cancer-causing agents in the environment. Some cancer activists of color discuss risk factors of breast cancer that are passionately disregarded by white cancer activists, but at least these risk factors give individuals a sense of control.

Presenting issues

Messages of activism must be presented broadly enough to reflect different societal conditions of various groups, but they must also speak visually to a diverse population. Within AIDS activism, prevention messages are distributed in different languages—mostly Spanish—and depict pictures of both non-white and white people. One activist within the AIDS movement who is also familiar with the breast cancer movement compares the AIDS movement to the breast cancer movement from the perspective of lesbians:

> There is not one perspective or one experience as a lesbian. . . . But what I do want to make up for [within AIDS activism] is the lack of what I consider to be fundamental voices in the dialogue of what our histories have been and our experiences are. When you don't have those stories, you can't draw a map that actually begins to trace the outlines that really reflect a diversity of experience because you don't have the stories, you don't have the histories or the perspectives that are lived experiences that people draw from to say this is what matters to me and this is what doesn't. And you also create an activism based on it because you are, again, lacking in the engines that start to be turned on by a different key. [A black poor lesbian] is not gonna be turned on by a breast cancer movement unless she would get breast cancer, but I mean in general that is not a movement that visually looks

inviting to her, that appears to be articulate about her life experience, talks about health in a way that she has experienced health issues. So even she has known, well, I don't want to have breast cancer, it would not necessarily be a place where she would see herself becoming an activist. The HIV movement, because it has been, because it is about poverty, a lot of it is about class and poverty. A lot of it is about the most vulnerable who are the most at risk around immediate health care. [AIDS movement]

At present, a poor black lesbian mother is not visually attracted to join breast cancer activism, because the breast cancer movement uses the symbols, icons, and language of a white middle-class and highly educated population. Although the disease has affected many celebrities of different ethnicities and sexual orientations who are potentially available to the cancer movement, many have chosen not to become involved. Here the breast cancer movement differs from the AIDS movement: because of the differences in the two diseases, the AIDS movement lacks celebrity spokeswomen who are HIV-positive.[16]

Nevertheless, despite their position to raise awareness through celebrity status spokeswomen with cancer, the existing grassroots cancer organizations have used Rachel Carson as an icon to express the movement's commitment to finding the environmental links of cancer. Carson was the author of the groundbreaking book *Silent Spring*, which uncovered the dangers of pesticides and is still considered a pioneering work and the spark that set off the environmental movement.[17] While Carson died of breast cancer in 1964, she is believed to have kept silent about her diagnosis in order to be perceived as an objective scientist.[18]

Instead of the white middle-class icon Rachel Carson,[19] diverse, high-profile women who have status within the lesbian community and communities of color could have been chosen. For example, in her book on African-American women and breast cancer, Sylvia Dunnavant pays tribute to Minnie Ripperton: "Minnie Ripperton, jazz singer, wife and mother had had a radical mastectomy" in the 1970s and was outspoken and active about the disease. Ripperton "traveled the country urging women to learn about early detection methods and prompt treatment. In 1977, as a result of her courageous efforts, she received the American Cancer Society's Courage Award from former President Jimmy Carter, the Ebony Music Ebby Award, and the NAACP Image Award."[20]

Many women with cancer are well-known figures in communities of color and in the lesbian community. Despite this, the cancer movement rarely mentions or pays tribute to them. I am often surprised by how little the cancer movement refers to Audre Lorde, who was a pioneer for cancer activism.[21] While the lesbian community pays regular tribute to Lorde and other women who have fallen prey to cancer,[22] the cancer movement neglects to honor this pioneer in cancer awareness. Evoking Lorde also helps bridge the white middle-class heterosexual cancer movement with communities of color and the lesbian community.[23] Overall, the AIDS movement uses celebrities more successfully as icons that can speak to a more diverse community.[24]

Resources for activism

A multicultural organizing style appears easier in the AIDS movement than in the cancer movement, partly due to the difference in financial resources available. That multicultural activism depends on financial resources has been determined by movements other than AIDS and breast cancer. Within the environmental justice movement, for instance, one insight gained after years of multicultural organizing is this:

> Multiracial organizing is more expensive than monoracial organizing. If we have any hope of keeping our organizations alive, everybody in the organization has to be trained and willing to raise resources, whether cash or in-kind. Some of our biggest expenses went into supporting an organizational structure in which different sorts of people could be active. They include paying licensed professionals to create a child care program, buying translation machines, training and paying translators, purchasing vans for transportation, and buying food.[25]

The breast cancer movement consists mainly of advocacy organizations that may offer support groups, but the movement lacks the necessary financial resources to provide direct services, education, and the like. As a result, there is an almost completely racially segregated activism in which white middle-class women with resources are engaged in grassroots cancer activism, but in which many women of color are associated with the affluent American Cancer Society.[26] One breast cancer activist of color addresses the economic imbalance between her community and white activism:

> I was approached once to collaborate with them [white grassroots cancer organization]. If you don't give me some funding for me to collaborate with you or to give my volunteers, I am not gonna, I am really not [going to] collaborate with you, as much as I would like to. Because my community has a lot of economic problems and I try to be sensitive to that. Voluntarism just for the heck of it, just for helping, it's not something that's very popular. I am not telling you that some people don't do it, some people do it. But the people do it because they have resources. You know, or they are getting something back. But generally Latinos have a lot of problems and I can't ask them to come to [location] to [travel] to pay for it, you know. To take a training that's not gonna be in Spanish. You know what I am saying, they need to be more sensitive to people's needs before they can say, I want to reach that community. Show me that you really want to reach that community. You know, come to my neighborhood as opposed to me coming to you. [cancer movement, woman of color]

On the other hand, resources are not a solution in themselves. If ideologies about race, sexuality, and class accept racial segregation as the norm in U.S. society, and further reinforce normative statuses such as being white, heterosexual, and middle class, even increased resources will not create any change. Ideology determines the distribution of resources. Within the AIDS movement, ideological practices have been documented by Nancy Stoller, who has studied the educational AIDS prevention material of two AIDS organizations, the San Francisco AIDS Foundation and New York City ACT UP.[27] Her findings indicate that

> the organizational cultures of both groups accept (or tolerate) American racial dominance patterns, including contemporary associations between racial and sexual behavior. In addition, decision-making processes in both organizations foster maintenance of racial domination by giving the greatest weight to white values.[28]

In addition to Stoller's warnings about the dangers of ideological practices, a second danger arises when large amounts of money are at a movement's disposal. Contributions from profit-driven sponsors are often not easily aligned with a movement's goals. The acceptance of outside support is one identity practice that also expresses the movement's collective identity.

AIDS activism is a good example that illustrates a potential conflict between the movement's collective identity of anti-classism and anti-racism and the identity practice of drawing in the support of profit-driven pharmaceutical industries.[29] While resources are needed to enable education or services, the intersection of the money-making interests of the pharmaceutical industry and the goals of AIDS activists is not without conflict. One activist who is critical of an alliance between pharmaceutical industry and AIDS activism argues that the industry's agenda prevails over the activists' interests in prolonging lives.

> I think there is an unholy alliance between AIDS activists and drug companies, so that some of this stuff is to put pressure and push, push, push and to get more drugs. But, on the other hand, the drug companies really call the shots. They fly in AIDS activists to conferences in a fancy hotel and wine and dine them and put them up on platforms to speak to doctors. There are AIDS activists who do circuits and have nice cocktail parties. It's just a different feel. Like no one ever did that in the civil rights movement, took a bunch of African Americans and flew them around the country to educate the races. You know, it's just a different world. There is a funny thing going on with the drug companies that makes me very uncomfortable. And there are also odd things going on with the sort of concept of empowerment, consumer empowerment. [AIDS movement]

Obviously a careful and critical analysis is needed to prevent the movement from falling into the trap of retarding its goals of anti-racism and anti-classism. If the pharmaceutical industry's ideological thinking prevails over the movement's collective identity of anti-classism and anti-racism, a situation may be created in which people's value and expendability are established according to the capitalist competitive market model.[30] As a result, people's well-being may be sacrificed, and human beings may be used toward certain ends that they may not be expecting.

> It's all about money. It's a money-making business now. It's a money-making business on people, and that's why I am really

reluctant to talk to a lot of people about what appalls me. It's because HIV-positive folks are being used like vouchers—serious vouchers to abuse HIV-positive people to get information and it's not fair. [AIDS movement, HIV-positive]

Building alliances

The alliances and coalitions that a movement builds are at the third layer of collective identity. It is not surprising that a movement's organizing style, presentation, and framing of issues are reflected and reinforced on the solidary level of collective identity as well.

I have presented a white heterosexual middle-class activism style as being dominant within the cancer movement.[31] Closest to the cancer movement are the environmental and women's movements. These allies tend to be similar in their class and racial makeup and in their prioritizing of a white, middle-class agenda. An orientation toward these two movements reinforces and maintains the already existing white middle-class culture of the cancer movement.

The cancer movement is working on coalition building with the environmental movement and especially women-dominated environmental organizations. This choice reinforces the existence of a white heterosexual middle-class culture within the cancer movement, since it is also the culture of the environmental movement.[32] While the cancer movement faces external sexism, the environmental movement has to deal with both external and internal sexism. Within the anti-toxins movement, which is the most radical wing of the environmental movement, considerable effort is being spent on confronting male chauvinism and instead integrating women's liberation and environmentalism.[33]

In 1991, with the emergence of the environmental justice movement, the whiteness of the environmental movement was challenged to reconstitute an environmental movement as more than just a white movement.[34] Some of the obstacles the environmental movement faces while attempting to include anti-racism into environmentalism are similar to those in the cancer movement. For instance, in the environmental movement, argues Robert Gottlieb, professionalization and Washington-focused lobbying efforts are barriers to a social justice dimension of environmental problems that incorporate race, gender, and class.[35] This applies to the cancer movement similarly in that the scientific objective framing of cancer is a barrier to an integration of diverse women who have other needs and demands. A culturally integrated approach to breast cancer activism has to take on a different agenda to accommodate the issues that are meaningful to the lives of women of color. Among others, the issues are socioeconomic and poverty concerns, housing, language barriers, and health access. One woman of color talked about conditions that shape the lives of women of color and prevent them from getting health care and treatment for breast cancer.

> The number one priority is family and children. A lot of the people in this community are the older women. Women that are in the risk group, which are older women are primary providers, either for their grandchildren or just their nieces, nephews, you know, whoever, somebody's kids. Somebody had a problem with substance abuse and rocked off and left the kid, and this older person takes them in. So that is very common here. We even have like grandmother's groups now and they are really strong women. To talk to them about breast cancer, they don't want to hear it. They don't want to hear it because if they get breast cancer, what's gonna happen to these kids who have been abandoned and put in their care for as-sistance? If they'll die and they'll feel like they are gonna die if they get breast cancer, what's gonna happen to these kids who trusted them to take care of them because they were abandoned? So they don't have time to look for a breast can-cer and they are afraid to find it even if it is there. They shut their eyes if they don't see it, it ain't there. So they let it go. [cancer movement, woman of color]

Some women-dominated environmental organizations with which the breast cancer movement works take a feminist stand that is best described as heterosexist.[36] The "Women and Life on Earth" conference was the inauguration of ecofeminism in the 1980s. Then it was con-cluded that, as mothers, nurturers, and caretakers, women should direct their creative energies to heal the planet,[37] again reinforcing the cancer movement's own feminist heterosexist culture. However, among the multitude of environmental organizations, groups such as "Women's Voices for the Earth" also exist. This organization states "that for significant environmental protection and social change to take place, the environmental movement must include and empower all sectors of the population, regardless of race, religion, economic status, sexual orienta-tion, or gender."[38] A detailed analysis of the environmental justice movement is needed to assess this movement's collective identity by examining its identity practices in terms of gender, race, class, and sexuality. It is beyond the scope of my analysis to determine whether expressions of diversity with regard to gender, race, class, and sexuality are limited to an ideological vision of inclusivity or are reflected in the movement's culture as well.

Finally, in addition to environmental organizations, which are the cancer movement's ally, the movement's proximity to the women's movement and the women's health movement have already been mentioned.[39] The cancer movement shares with the women's movement a version of feminism that prioritizes gender oppression over other forms of oppression. The women's movement—largely a white middle-class one—shares this background with the cancer movement. Moreover, the feminist agenda has been largely determined by the issues and demands of white, middle-class women. Barbara Ryan argues that:

> Feminist goals such as ERA, abortion, child care, parental leave, and affirmative action are generalizable across populations, those gains that have been made in career and economic advance have benefited white middle-class women to a much greater extent than poor women and women of color.[40]

That the women's movement has embraced cancer rather than AIDS is therefore not surprising. Cancer fits comfortably into a feminist agenda that prioritizes the needs of white middle-class women, whereas AIDS does not.[41] Women of color have criticized the women's movement for not addressing issues that are central to their life conditions: welfare, public housing, tenants' rights, inner-city schools, poverty, drugs, racist rates of imprisonment, unemployment, and underemployment.[42] Most of these issues that are neglected by the women's movement are also central to AIDS activism. One AIDS activist talks about the silence of the women's movement in the 1980s, when more women became infected and affected by HIV:

> The reason that the women's movement hadn't taken it on was class and race. If you actually look at the feminist movement and *Ms.* magazine, the media attention, and then the internal organizing coming out of the National Organization of Women and a variety of kind of more established women's organizations, they never raised HIV as an issue. It was never part of their agenda. [AIDS movement]

The perception of the women's movement's definition of feminism as one that denies the importance of issues that are central in AIDS activism is common among AIDS activists. While women AIDS activists are feminists and would like to build coalitions with the women's movement, this would require the women's movement to include issues of poverty, race, class, and sexual orientation, which are the central issues to women and HIV.

> You know, some time it's very easy to be a feminist, if you are better off, you know. And sometimes not even not looking at the situation that other women are living in. Sometimes thinking why change their situation, they are poor, or because they have less resources, even though, I personally support the feminist movement. But what I am trying to say is that we need to learn how to work better with each other. [AIDS movement]

The AIDS movement is more closely aligned with the gay and lesbian movement than with the women's movement, and the contrary is true for the cancer movement. First, the AIDS movement's alliance with the gay and lesbian movement stems from the appearance of AIDS in the gay male community. Second, a number of AIDS organizations have emerged that were founded by gays and lesbians and are still rooted within the gay community. The alliance between gays and lesbians and AIDS is based on a male perspective. The existing overlap between homophobia and more general issues of sexuality binds the AIDS and the gay and lesbian movements together to this day.

With the exception of lesbian cancer organizations, the cancer movement does not reach out to the gay and lesbian movement. The gay and lesbian movement, however, frequently integrates breast cancer in its agenda. For instance, gay and lesbian events, such as gay pride, emphasize the importance of AIDS and breast cancer as though these were the only two health concerns of the gay and lesbian community. Gay and lesbian support of breast cancer activism is also expressed in regard to fund-raising. Lesbians raise funds for specific and national cancer organizations. The non-profit organization Rainbow Endowment,[43] for example, distributes its funds to gay and lesbian organizations as well as to organizations active in breast cancer and AIDS.[44] One activist who favors a broader, more inclusive gay and lesbian health agenda speaks to the presentation of AIDS and breast cancer as though they were the diseases of the gay and lesbian community:

There is a kind of ideological line drawn as though it were real: there are lesbians with breast cancer and there are gay men with HIV. Those are the two big queer health movements. . . . I have been able to . . . work to build a lesbian health movement that doesn't articulate one health agenda over another, doesn't privilege one over the other, but says, there is a lesbian health agenda and access issues that look different for women depending on what their backgrounds are, what their ages are, what their sexual orientation is, that all of those are the factors that we have to look at when we are facing life-challenging crises rather than there is a lesbian breast cancer movement and then there is a gay HIV movement and that was really how it was seen. [AIDS movement]

These differences between the breast cancer and AIDS movements in regard to alliances reinforce the existing internal conditions of each movement. That is, a movement that has a white middle-class, heterosexist culture as the cancer movement uses identity practices of framing and presenting its agenda from a particular perspective but, in addition, it also draws on movements and allies that stem from and fit within the white middle-class, heterosexist perspective. The AIDS movement, on the other hand, has a broader definition of issues, since it struggles with the problems of sexism, homophobia, racism, poverty, and classism.

In this chapter, the AIDS and breast cancer movements have been discussed according to the broadness of their vision and their identity practices as expressed in movement culture, organizational structure, and outside support and resources. Solidary with other movements, the third layer in which collective identity is embedded has been shown to reinforce a movement's collective identity. Hence, a movement's collective identity of diversity is reflected in all layers, from the individual movement organization to the movement and its allies. When one applies the concept of identity practices, one can evaluate a movement's collective identity, by inquiring about its identity practices that express and reflect the movement's collective identity.

CHAPTER 7

Conclusion

This chapter discusses the findings of the comparison between activists involved in the AIDS and breast cancer movements. Throughout this book, the similarities and differences between activists from these two movements have been highlighted. Within this chapter, these similarities and differences are put into the context of lessons that are informative to other social change activists and sociologists.

Motivating people to activism

Women activists in the AIDS and breast cancer movements have been motivated by personal and political reasons. This knowledge offers an important insight for social movement theorists and social change activists. It reveals that there are two conditions for motivation. Knowing about both conditions means that movements have some control over mobilizing and recruiting members. A movement can frame an issue by either personalizing or politicizing it, which gives its organizers control. Many questions arise then, including the following: How does a movement know into what direction the movement should direct the issue? Do personalizing and politicizing work equally well? Are there ways in which a movement can determine whether its organizing issue should be predominantly personalized or predominantly politicized?

It is not arbitrary whether a movement puts the emphasis on personalizing or politicizing the issue around which it organizes. To motivate new members to activism, depending on the particular issue, one is more effective than the other. It depends on the issue itself whether the movement is more effective by personalizing or politicizing the issue.

AIDS and breast cancer activism suggests that there is an underlying rationale that makes either the personalizing or the politicizing of an issue more effective. Before the emergence of a movement, issues are already framed as either personal or public. I suggest that the effective technique for a movement is to put more emphasis on the opposite quality of the issue's initial framing. For instance, breast cancer was framed as a personal and private issue prior to the movement's emergence. Hence, an effective strategy for the cancer movement is to work more heavily on framing cancer politically. In the case of AIDS, the disease was public and political as soon as it emerged and before the emergence of an AIDS movement. AIDS was political because it was perceived as a menace to public safety and the lives and health of the "general population." So personalizing the issue by putting a human face on AIDS proved an effective strategy for motivating activism around this disease.

In support of the statement that the personalizing of AIDS was effective for activism, here are some of the battles the movement fought. There were many symbolic battles fought between AIDS activists and those controlling and administering AIDS. Many battles were fought in the context of medicine and law that claimed a unified and coherent tradition, but instead they divided individuals into conscious subjects—or embodied subjects versus mere bodies, as Susan Bordo argues.[1] Bordo's analysis of such double standards in medicine and law reveals the social practice of dividing individuals into two groups: those who occupy the cultural location of subjects and those who are "others." The one group with subject status has protection from the individual right of bodily integrity, whereas the other group has been "denied those protections, becoming for all medical and legal purposes pure *res extensa*, bodies stripped of their animating, dignifying, and humanizing 'subject-ivity.' "[2] That people with AIDS were perceived by the societal powers as "others" or "bodies stripped of subjectivity" was expressed in many ways. For instance, attempts to implement mandatory testing, the treatment of HIV-positive women and HIV-positive mothers, and the treatment of HIV-positive women and pregnancy all indicate the "othering" of these groups.

Other examples taken from the AIDS discourse show that early on the AIDS movement fought a battle over the naming of the issue. AIDS activists argued in favor of labeling those afflicted by the disease "people with AIDS," whereas the other side talked about "AIDS victims." "People with AIDS" is personal in that it gives subjectivity to and maintains the personhood of those with the disease. Victims of a disease, however, are the faceless, nameless thousands who are merely bodies.

Similarly, the AIDS Quilt makes the disease visible and personal. The Quilt does more than express the memory of those who have lost a loved one; it also gives other people, whether they have or have not known people with AIDS, a personal connection to AIDS. One practice within the AIDS movement provides another example: the phrase of those "infected and those affected by AIDS" unites people with and without the disease. Further, it personalizes the issue in that it creates a personal relationship to AIDS for everyone. These examples illustrate how the movement personalized the disease and maintained the personhood and subjectivity of those with AIDS. It worked against the societal powers that had been intended to deprive people with AIDS of their dignity and the protection of their individual rights.

In contrast, cancer has always been perceived as a personal and private disease. Further, the subjectivity of people with cancer has not been challenged as with AIDS.[3] As long as cancer was perceived as a personal issue, it lacked conflict and insurgency. The conflict arose as soon as early cancer activists laid the groundwork for a movement response to the disease through the presentation of a political framing of cancer. Among others, these political messages were that research on women's health is underfunded, that research on cancer prevention is underfunded, and that cancer is dominated by the economic interests of the cancer industry and its gender dynamics. Such politicization of a previously private and personal disease was an effective strategy. The movement's politicization of cancer, by pointing to the societal neglect of women's health and the sexism that dominates medicine, was an effective strategy for activism. Furthermore, the cancer movement's existing political agenda should be expanded by demanding societal change in health care—that is, universal health care availability so that cancer screening and treatment are available equally to all groups and survival times and mortality rates are no longer correlated to race and income. A part of this agenda, of course, is knowing and studying how and why cancer affects different populations, such as lesbians and women of color.

Hence, findings taken from the AIDS and cancer movements indicate that a movement's success depends on invoking the countermessage in addition to the existing framing of an issue as either personal or political. Activism demands that both a personal framing and a political framing of issues have to be present so people are motivated. In that sense, the awareness of an issue's societal perception before a movement's emergence informs and guides the movement's frame. A movement that emphasizes the issue's counterpoint increases the potential for motivation to activism by providing a possible constituency with both personal and political links to the issue.

My model argues that creating personal and political links to issues informs social movements about effective strategies. For instance, the history of the gay and lesbian movement supports this model. The history of the movement indicates that it put forward a political framing of gay and lesbian issues when such issues were traditionally perceived as private ones. Moreover, knowing the conditions that motivate activism offers sociologists a model for predicting movement emergence. In that sense, having a model for motivation is a helpful tool for sociologists and movement activists. But social reality is complex, and it is therefore too simplistic and mechanical to assume that a movement will be immediately effective if it emphasizes the counterpoint to an issue's societal perception before movement emergence.

Activism's intersection with gender, race, class, and sexuality

Interviews with one gender group, women activists, are the basis for this model. We have seen that women are motivated to activism by a personal and political relationship to the issue. The women who had this relationship were of color, white, poor, affluent, lesbian, and straight women. These findings are not readily applicable to men, and it is even less clear how men's motivations intersect with race, class, and sexual orientation. Men may be motivated by different conditions than both the personal and political described here. One could argue that motivational conditions are different for men because some women who participate in AIDS activism do so because a male friend has contracted HIV. In contrast, there is no similar motivational response from men within the cancer movement. Husbands, male lovers, fathers, brothers, and friends seem not to feel equally compelled to become active.[4] In terms of sexuality, straight men are generally not associated with AIDS activism, and the cancer movement appears to be without gay and straight men. This is one indicator that motivations to activism might differ depending on gender and sexuality. Men who have higher status in society seem not to be motivated to become active on behalf of women, as women's issues such as breast cancer and pro-choice activism indicate. However, women who have less power and status can be motivated to become active on behalf of privileged men.

This difference becomes even more prominent if one takes into account the emergence of men's health organizations and prostate cancer organizations in particular. Men did not become active in support of women; instead, they took breast cancer as a model for activism and focused on their issues. In 1990, prostate cancer patients in Chicago founded "US TOO," an organization named in direct response to breast cancer activism.[5] One major goal of US TOO is to use political advocacy to reach the same kind of funding as AIDS and breast cancer.[6] More organizing followed. In 1991, the Men's Health Network Coalition was founded. This organization defines itself as "an informational and educational organization recognizing men's health as a specific social concern and committed to promoting issues affecting men's health."[7] In 1996, a national organization, the National Prostate Cancer Coalition, was launched, which describes itself as "a dynamic coalition of individuals and organizations dedicated to the fight for increased funding for prostate cancer research that will lead to a cure."[8]

Contrary to women's breast cancer organizations, health activism by men solicits women's support. The Men's Health Network Coalition states:

> Our goal is to focus media attention on problems which plague men and which, by extension, affect the women in their lives. By achieving this goal, we will sensitize the public to the health care problems of men and the unfortunate effects those problems have on their loved ones, their employers, and our health care infrastructure.[9]

Similarly, US TOO launched US TOO Partners in 1998.[10] This support network for partners of prostate cancer patients defines prostate cancer as a family disease that affects women who then have the opportunity to find support by joining women's self-help groups called US TOO Partners. This type of organizing shows the absence of awareness about sexual orientation in this movement's discourse by operating in a heterosexist framework. Further, the prostate cancer organizations' solicitation of women appears to point to an interesting gender differ-ence in the targeted constituency. Hence, how men's motivation to ac-tivism intersects with race, class, and sexuality and what kind of effect this has on social movements are important areas of inquiry for future research.[11]

Different social conditions

After having analyzed motivation to activism, I remind readers that breast cancer activists operate in a different context than do women AIDS activists. Earlier, the differential context of both health crises was discussed. There was a high incidence of breast cancer among white middle-class women, whereas poor and low-income women of color have a higher incidence of AIDS. The same incidence is believed to exist concerning sexual orientation.[12] Lesbians are assumed to be at low risk for HIV but at high risk for breast cancer. Such differences regarding sexual orientation and racial and socioeconomic background make for an altered social context for activism and a different societal perception of both diseases.

Further, the historical context is different insofar as the AIDS movement emerged in the early 1980s, whereas grassroots breast can-cer organizations emerged roughly 10 years later, thus the movements have existed for different lengths of time. For this research, however, the interviews with women activists took place at the same time with women who are currently active in either movement. The time gap between each movement's emergence provides activists with a differ-ent social context. The length of time for which each movement has existed shapes the social context of AIDS or breast cancer activism differently. More specifically, these two movements are in different stages of mobilization.[13]

Stages of mobilization

In the last fifteen years, the AIDS movement not only was able to sustain itself, but it also changed and expanded. In that sense, it has to be perceived as more mature and mobilized than the younger breast cancer movement.

Social movement theorists have documented the life of social movements beginning with movement emergence. The recent grassroots cancer movement is an example of this process.[14] The orga-nizing of activists around breast cancer in the 1990s brought breast cancer as a political issue into public awareness. In return, this caused more women to become conscious of breast cancer activism and to be drawn into the movement. On the one hand, such a response leads to an increase in movement members. On the other hand, it brings together a mix of activist cohorts with different backgrounds regarding organizing and political consciousness. Social movement theorist Nancy Whittier calls these phases of expansion "transition periods."[15] According to Whittier, a transition period is marked by the entry of a new political cohort of activists that differs from the current political cohort. The melting together of different political cohorts is a process in which the definition of the movement's collective identity is challenged and renegotiated. Whittier states:

> As larger numbers of recruits enter a movement, assuming leadership positions in preexisting movement organizations or establishing new groups, they attempt to reformulate organizational goals and strategies, ideological interpretations, and movement culture. These changes, not surprisingly, produce intergenerational conflict. Yet, in order for a movement to shift to a higher level of mobilization, new participants must enter. The passing of social movements from one political generation to another thus becomes the key to movement survival over the long haul.[16]

With regard to the AIDS movement, its fifteen years of existence indicate that it has witnessed several generations of AIDS activists who have sustained the movement. The AIDS movement is a more developed, more mobilized one compared to the more recent, less mobilized cancer movement. "More mobilized" describes a movement that has reached a more advanced stage of mobilization. Evolution from less mobilized to more mobilized occurs when a movement becomes more complex in its collective identity. Such complexity evolves from what Whittier calls "transition periods." This progression from less mobilized to more mobilized is not caused by the amount of time for which a movement has existed or the number of people involved, but there are of course correlations between time and number of people. A movement that has existed longer and has involved more people has a likelihood of having undergone several transitions that have led to a more mobilized situation.

Being able to distinguish these two movements in regard to their stages of mobilization is an important outcome of the comparison of women AIDS and breast cancer activists. At the outset of this study, I anticipated finding differences between women AIDS and women cancer activists. It was not possible, however, to foresee that differences between these two groups of women would stem from different stages of mobilization. Differences between women AIDS and cancer activists are expressions of activism in different stages of mobilization, which can now be discussed systematically as indicators of a more developed or less developed stage of mobilization.

Use of resources

When they organize for social change, social movements depend on resources. The activists of the AIDS and cancer movements are no exception. Both movements have activists who have political experience and organizing skills and use their expertise to the movement's benefit.[17] Both movements accomplished the activation of new resources, such as encouraging formerly inactive women to participate in the movements. One commonality that has been presented between these first-time AIDS and breast cancer activists is their usage of "personal resources" for AIDS and cancer activism. First-time cancer activists use resources that are available to them, usually resources that stem from privilege—these available to white middle-class women. Such resources are education, income, sense of empowerment and entitlement, and access to influential institutions and powerful people in politics or the health field. While this type of resources is used in AIDS activism[18] as well, first-time women AIDS activists offer another set of resources—the resources of marginality. In other words, first-time women AIDS activists principally use "marginality resources" such as various forms of survival skills developed through living as disadvantaged persons, including women of color, lesbians, prostitutes, ex-offenders, IV-drug users, and poor people.

That the AIDS movement is more mobilized suggests the following about the relationship between resources and mobilization: the more mobilized a movement is, the more diverse the resources that are used by its activists. This rule gives social movement theorists and social change activists valuable information about movements. It indicates that a more highly mobilized movement draws on a more diverse constituency because more resources are accessed and made available by a heterogeneous constituency. Social movement theorists who pay close attention to the resources used by a particular movement can use this information to evaluate a movement's stage of mobilization. Social change activists who are concerned about their movement's success and sustainability should take a critical look at their movement's resources in regard to their homogeneity. Such awareness allows activists to work toward a higher level of mobilization by bringing in new and different resources for their movement. Diversifying a movement's resources requires that it broaden its constituency. After all, resources are tied to people, and diverse people possess different resources.

Recruitment of constituency

Social movement literature identifies at least three different agents for recruitment: existing organizations, individual activists, and contact with the role of activist and immersion in the movement's subculture.[19] Most important among these recruitment processes are the existing organizations and social networks that can be used as building blocks for social movements. Social movement literature argues that recruiting members of existing organizations and social networks is an effective form of gaining supporters for social movements.[20] One of the main advantages of this type of recruitment is that it is less time consuming than, for instance, interactions between individual activists and potential recruits. This most effective form of recruitment, the merging between organizations and the building of alliances with other organizations, can, however, have a constraining or an enabling effect on the mobilization of diverse populations with diverse resources. For instance, an alliance between a predominantly white cancer movement and a predominantly white environmental organization does not diversify either movement's constituency or resources, it merely increases the number of involved people who are supportive of the issue. In contrast, a movement's decision to allocate time and energy to the building of alliances with a racially, sexually, and otherwise different organization could be an effective means of diversifying a movement's constituency. For instance, the AIDS movement initially relied heavily on recruiting members of the gay and lesbian community, but today that movement is more diversified. Hence, in the AIDS movement's more developed stage of mobilization, the gay and lesbian community is no longer the exclusive pool for recruiting activists. Instead, AIDS activists come from a range of organizational backgrounds, from political organizations to service organizations, unions, and churches. To absorb activists from such diverse backgrounds, a movement has to have a multitude of social movement organizations that speak to activists with different organizational histories. The structure of a more mobilized movement shows a multitude of diversified movement organizations that support activists with different histories, goals, and strategies. The less mobilized cancer movement has yet to achieve a structure that validates different activists by providing them with a variety of movement organizations with different strategies and goals.

The organizational style with which the movement operates is an intrinsic part of recruitment. The recruiting and organizing practices used for different constituencies need to be sensitive to race, class, and sexuality. Various cultural differences have to be taken into account when the goal of a movement is to approach different communities. To be successful, recruiting and organizing have to be filtered with respect to race, class, and sexuality. For instance, Prudence Posner writes, "Organizing in African-American neighborhoods cannot be understood as simply organizing with a black face,"[21] and Latina activists point out that there are distinct cultural obstacles in communities to the white middle-class style of organizing. This shows that more mobilized, more evolved movements are multidimensional in every way—their constituency, their resources, their organizing styles, and their recruitment techniques. Less mobilized movements tend to be narrower and might even be one-dimensional. The most important process that guides a movement toward achieving multiplicity and essentially a more evolved stage of mobilization is the movement's collective identity.

Construction of collective identity

A movement's collective identity is the outcome of a process, and the identity is not static. Nancy Whittier argues:

> In the process of constructing a collective identity, challenging groups adopt labels for themselves [such as AIDS and cancer activists], draw lines between insiders and outsiders, and develop interpretive frameworks, a political consciousness through which members understand the world. Of course, "collective identities" exist only as far as real people agree upon, enact, argue over, and internalize them; group definitions have no life of their own, and they are constantly changing rather than static.[22]

Whether a movement is more mobilized and therefore more diverse and complex is reflected in its collective identity. A movement that is becoming more mobilized will refine its collective identity to reflect its increasing diversity. But the diversity reflected in a movement's collective identity is more complex than the sum of its diverse groups. The task of the collective identity is to bridge gaps between different groups.

The job of tying together different groups is difficult and dangerous. Social movement theorist Alberto Melucci points to one possible danger—"integralism." That is, the "yearning for a totalizing identity, for a 'masterkey which unlocks every door of reality.' Integralism, says Melucci, rejects a pluralist and 'disenchanted' attitude to life and encourages people to 'turn their backs on complexity' and become incapable of recognizing difference."[23] This sets up an all too familiar dilemma for movements. On the one hand, diversifying is important with respect to mobilization. On the other hand, as Melucci warns, a totalizing collective identity applicable to any constituency could diminish the real differences between groups. If this is so, how do movements handle differences?

Activists within a movement have to walk the thin line of uniting people based on their common grievances (such as AIDS and breast cancer) while acknowledging the groups' particularities. For an achievement of this balancing act, movement activists' perception of the world must be flexible and must encompass an understanding of the specific issues of AIDS and breast cancer and include, among others, racism, sexism, classism, heterosexism, and ableism. Based on my comparative analysis of AIDS and breast cancer activists, this balancing act is further developed in more mobilized movements. Less mobilized movements have yet to work on the transformative consciousness[24] that is needed for performing this balancing act. The straight woman AIDS activist who is knowledgeable about discrimination based on sexual orientation and the affluent gay male activist who stands up for a straight IV-drug woman user is the prototype of transformed consciousness.

The most important requirement for the achievement of such transformation is communication. Communication within a movement must be open about the existence of differences. For activists coming from different backgrounds, an understanding of differences requires that movement discourse must provide information about these differences and their effects on people's lives. The cancer movement has yet to reach open communication about differences. Its glossing over differences will not create the transformation of consciousness that is needed for reaching a more mobilized stage. The cancer movement's discourse of "we are all women" does not take into account that women's life situations are different, depending on whether we are lesbians or straight, rich or poor, or white or of color. Hence, many cancer activists are lacking information about the reality of women who are different than they. In that sense, the cancer movement has yet to expand the participant activists' worldviews so that they understand that cancer is played out differently between poor and affluent women.

The glossing over of differences between women that cancer activists employ brings what Charlotte Ryan calls "quick victories."[25] The price for pursuing these quick victories is that the transformation of activists' worldviews is neglected. Instead, as long as activists stay involved in the movement, the necessary education about racism, sexism, classism, heterosexism, and the like will spontaneously occur as a by-product of activism. Some think it is sufficient, however, for people to work together on one issue, and that it is of lesser importance that people have different worldviews aside from that one issue.

Developing a strategy for the long haul

Many activist theorists have made important arguments against the pursuit of quick victories. Instead, these activists argue for long-term strategies. Remaining aware of long-term goals requires activists to undergo the painstaking process of acknowledging and addressing differences. It means taking the time to negotiate differences and working on a broader frame—a collective identity that encompasses the particularities of different groups in relation to the issue of resurgency. What does such collective identity look like?

Identity construction is difficult. Even before the collective level, many discuss difficulties of constructing individual identities. Difficulties on the individual level are a fragmentation of the self or a separation of one's multiple identities that reduces the multiplicity of identities to a singular one. For instance, Gloria Anzaldua asks:

> What am I? *A third world lesbian feminist with Marxist and mystic leanings.* They would chop me up into little fragments and tag each piece with a label. [emphasis in original][26]

Similarly, Audre Lorde expresses her vision of embracing differences and using them to nourish movements. She states:

> You do not have to be me in order for us to fight alongside each other. I do not have to be you to recognize that our wars are the same. What we must do is commit ourselves to some future that can include each other and to work toward that future with the particular strengths of our individual identities. And in order to do this, we must allow each other our differences at the same time we recognize our sameness. If our history has taught us anything, it is that action for change directed only against the external conditions of our oppressions is not enough.[27]

Difference needs to be embraced when different people are fighting for a common goal. Social movement theorists are also uttering similar statements. They suggest that the bridging of differences between previously segregated social groups accounts in part for the cultural impact of a social movement.[28] Moreover, social movement theorists state that creating an environment (community) within a movement that is already operating according to its vision of a liberated world with egalitarian contact between groups is an important task.[29] A movement's struggle for social change takes a long time, but, while in the midst of this struggle, important steps can be made toward creating a "better world" within a movement.

June Jordan points to the reality of working in a movement and to the potential limitations of social movements' ability to create a community between different people:

> It occurs to me that much organizational grief could be avoided if people understood that partnership in misery does not necessarily provide for partnership for change: When we get the monsters off our backs all of us may want to run in very different directions.[30]

Hence, the creation of a collective identity that is broad enough to reflect different groups and unite them is the most central task of social movements. All along, social movement theorists have argued that constructing a collective identity is central to social movements.[31] I expand on this by stating that constructing a broader collective identity is central to evolving into advanced mobilization.

Further, a broader frame or collective identity eases the building of alliances and assists in moving toward a more mobilized stage.

Solidarity with a movement is more easily established if, for example, the cancer movement's collective identity reflects the particular relationship to cancer of lesbians and women of color. By organizing around cancer through the lenses of gender, class, race, and sexual orientation, the less mobilized cancer movement is more likely to appeal to a diverse constituency and to draw some of them in as members. So the cancer movement could appeal to other movements or organizations that are already working on issues such as lesbian rights, economic justice, and environmental racism. This leads to a more evolved mobilizational stage and increases the movement's ability to sustain activism over the long haul.

In contrast to these arguments that are favorable to a broadening of the movement's framing of AIDS and breast cancer, it is important to show the limitations and downfalls of this approach. Social movement theorists Debra Friedman and Doug McAdam discuss the life of social movements as undergoing different stages. One of these stages regards retaining a movement's existing members and attracting new ones. They state that a counterintuitive process exists in that the movement's collective identity, which covers a wide range of issues, tends to make a movement more rather than less exclusive.

> [B]y extending the scope of its mission, an SMO [social movement organization] actually narrows the field of potential participants. When there are many attitudes and behavioral prescriptions associated with participation, it is more likely that attitude conflicts will exist between the prospective participants and the SMO. A broader conception may also lead to conflict within the organization itself. Social movement organizations that attempt to construct all-purpose collective identities may therefore appeal to a narrower audience than those that stand fast to a more limited conception.[32]

This seems to contradict all previous arguments in favor of diversity and a widening of activists' worldviews. That may not be necessarily so, but it points to some possible dangers. Opening up a movement's collective identity toward more inclusivity can potentially cause a movement's vision to become murky. The movement risks losing its clear boundaries and watering down the issue that initially caused an organizational response. Again, this stresses the difficult balancing act that a movement has to perform. It has to balance between being exclusive due to a narrow focus and being an all-purpose movement that is inclusive by adding on to the initial issue. For instance, a hypothetical breast cancer movement that raises awareness about cancer, fights for lesbians' rights to adopt and have custody of children, favors affirmative action, champions improved housing facilities for the poor, and supports new laws for the location of toxic waste facilities is truly unlikely to attract more members, because the movement attempts to solve everything. People interested in toxic waste sites are most likely more attracted to an anti-toxins movement that allows them to concentrate on environmental issues, but in this hypothetical cancer movement they would be required to give their attention to many other issues. Adding on issues is not what is meant by the broadening of a movement's collective identity to reflect diversity to be more compelling to a diverse constituency. The distinction between these two versions of inclusivity is that one treats diversity additively, by adding on more issues to the original cause, whereas the other type maintains the focus on the original issue but expands it to a more multilayered picture that reflects the issue through the lenses of race, class, gender, and sexuality.

Activists in the AIDS movement have a much broader perspective of AIDS in that they look at the disease from the perspectives of race, class, gender, and sexuality. A broadening of the collective identity through the use of different lenses unites different groups and makes the original issue such as AIDS or cancer a compelling one to many. A movement's collective identity broadens over time, as the AIDS movement has demonstrated, and it is a sign of an evolution to a more advanced stage of mobilization. The current breast cancer activism, however, has yet to broaden its frame to sustain its existing members and to gain more diverse ones.

This is certainly one possibility for the future of the breast cancer movement. The future of the AIDS and the breast cancer movements can hold a number of new challenges. The AIDS movement has been successful in broadening its collective identity and advancing to a more mobilized stage. But time will tell whether the AIDS movement will be able to maintain this level of mobilization. The recent, exciting medical advances of new drugs such as protease inhibitors, which radically improve the treatment of HIV/AIDS, create a new challenge for the AIDS movement. One outcome is that certain activism responses declined, such as monetary donations and participation in AIDS events and organizations. The new drugs are extremely costly, and they have changed HIV/AIDS from a terminal to a chronic disease. In general, 1996 was considered the turning point in the AIDS epidemic in that the effects of new treatments were reflected in national morbidity and mortality statistics. CDC data on U.S. deaths attributed to AIDS decreased by 42 percent between 1996 and 1997.[33] The decline in deaths, however, is greater among men than women and more prominent in whites and in men who have sex with men.[34] This points to crucial differences among persons with AIDS. There are those who can afford to pay for the drugs or who have access to drug treatment, and they are therefore in a much better position to prolong their lives. This poses a new challenge for AIDS activism. Under these changed conditions, will the movement be capable of sustaining a collective identity that looks at HIV/AIDS through the multilayered lens of race, class, gender, and sexuality? Or will AIDS activists regress to striving for quick victories? This conflict is not an easy one since, after all, the AIDS and cancer movements are both organized around a life-threatening disease.

The cancer movement could potentially be similarly challenged in the future. The media reports more and more often about important advancements in cancer research, for example, on substances that shrink tumors. While advances and success in cancer research are much needed, they could, however, lead to new dilemmas similar to the one faced in AIDS, that treatment benefits are unequal. Further, both movements are confronted with changes regarding health activism. The successes of AIDS activism triggered women to become active in the breast cancer movement. Then prostate cancer organizations emerged, and they were also successful in increasing prostate cancer funding and putting the spotlight on men's health problems. This points to the politicization of health and a previously unknown competition between diseases regarding resources such as media attention, activists, and research dollars. Diseases are pitted against each other, and there are no solutions about how to determine the "right" amount of spending on a disease. Competing criterion are suggested, such as spending on medical research should be determined by a dollars-per-death formula, whereas others argue that diseases that affect young people should be funded.[35] The politicization of health and such competing interests between disease advocates point to the complexity of health movements' task in defining their collective identities. They are also another reminder that collective identity is not static but instead needs constant renegotiation.

In conclusion, I have used some of the findings presented throughout this book and discussed them as lessons for social movement theorists and social change activists. Knowing that a personal and political link are necessary for turning people into activists is essential for sustaining both the AIDS and cancer movements. It also points to the outstanding accomplishments of AIDS and breast cancer activists. Cancer activists chose to politicize cancer in the same way in which AIDS activists personalized AIDS, which were successful strategies for breast cancer and AIDS activism. But the model of combining a personal and political link can also inform other social change activists. Further, being able to name indicators that are present at various stages of mobilization gives social movement theorists a framework for evaluating social movements in regard to the level of mobilization. Social change activists benefit from this knowledge in that it essentially provides them with a tool for moving their movement closer to a more evolved mobilizational stage and thereby closer to social change.

Appendix: Sample

I interviewed thirty-seven women. Nineteen were part of the cancer movement, and seventeen were part of the AIDS movement. One woman was part of both the AIDS movement and the cancer movement. Three women who were part of the cancer movement at the time of the interview had prior involvement in the AIDS movement.

Of the thirty-seven women, twenty were white and seventeen were of color. I interviewed twenty women without either disease and seventeen women with a disease. Of the seventeen women with a disease, seven were women with breast cancer, three were women with another type of cancer, and seven were women with HIV/AIDS. One of the women with HIV/AIDS also had a form of cancer before her HIV/AIDS diagnosis. Eighteen women described themselves as lesbians, seventeen described themselves as straight, and two women cancer activists stated personal reasons for not describing themselves with regard to sexual orientation. They explained that they had reasons to identify neither as lesbians nor as straight women, nor did they identify as bisexuals.

Ten interviewed women had no prior political experience, whereas twenty-seven women drew on a variety of political movements (e.g., labor, left, civil rights, anti-war, gay and lesbian, student, and Central American). Six women without prior political experience were part of the AIDS movement; the other four first-time activists were part of the cancer movement.

The interviewed AIDS activists were members of their organizations for an average of 6.4 years (a median of five years); the length of membership ranged from between six months and fourteen years. The interviewed cancer activists were involved in the cancer movement for 3.05 years (a median of three years); among the cancer activists, the length of membership ranged from 1.5 years to 5.5 years.

The age of the interviewed cancer activists ranged from twenty-eight to sixty-four. The average age of the interviewed cancer activists was forty-six. The age range for AIDS activists was twenty-five to fifty-nine. The average age of the interviewed activists was forty.

The class composition of the sample was based on the women's self-described class identity. That is, there were a number of women who had been raised working class and who self-identified as middle class. Other women had been raised working class and had maintained a working-class identity, even though they had an occupation that was considered middle class. Among the seventeen interviewed AIDS activists, ten women were working class or were raised poor. Of these ten women with a working-class or lower-class background, 3 said that they lead middle-class lives today. Seven AIDS activists were middle class. One woman said that she was raised lower middle class, and another woman said that she was raised upper middle class.

Of the twenty interviewed cancer activists, a majority of sixteen were middle class. Of these sixteen, one was raised upper middle class, one was raised upper middle class and is today middle class, 4 were raised poor or working class and are middle class today, and 4 more were raised lower middle class and are middle class today. Four interviewed women cancer activists had a working-class identity.

Notes

INTRODUCTION

1. Associated Press, "Breast Cancer Risk in Lesbians Put at 1 in 3," *Boston Globe* (February 5, 1993): 12.

CHAPTER 1

1. James T. Patterson, *The Dread Disease: Cancer and Modern American Culture* (Cambridge: Harvard University Press, 1987), 71.
2. Ibid, 72.
3. Sharon Batt, *Patient No More: The Politics of Breast Cancer* (Charlottetown, Canada: gynergy books, 1994), 295.
4. Reach to Recovery is a much criticized program. Briefly, it is a program that enlists volunteers to visit mastectomy patients in the hospital right after their surgery to give them temporary prostheses and offers advice about where to shop for a prosthesis, bathing suit, and so forth. Reach to Recovery has been criticized by many women because it operates in an oppressive gender framework. It needs perfect women, women with no visual signs of cancer, who will train other women to become perfect in hiding their mastectomies as well. Audre Lorde attacked this approach poignantly when she wrote, "Breast prostheses are offered to women after surgery in much the same way that candy is offered to babies after an injection, never mind that the end effect may be destructive. Their comfort is illusory." Audre Lord, *The Cancer Journals* (San Francisco: Aunt Lute, 1980), 64. Gender-oppressive thinking also inspired another activity of the ACS, the "Look Good Feel Better"

campaign. This program started in 1988 and is sponsored by cosmetics companies. It is available to women who are undergoing chemotherapy or radiation treatment. The women are taught how to use makeup and hair care techniques to hide visible signs of cancer, such as discoloration of the skin and hair loss. Sharon Batt, *Patient No More: The Politics of Breast Cancer* (Charlottetown, Canada: gynergy books, 1994). In Massachusetts, another similar program called "Beauty for Life" exists. According to the ACS informational brochure, it is a community-based breast cancer awareness partnership between the Massachusetts Cosmetology Association and the American Cancer Society.

Rose Kushner criticized the ACS as being male dominated in her groundbreaking book *Breast Cancer: A Personal History* in 1975. When she published the first edition of *Why Me? What Every Woman Should Know* in 1977, more women had been added to the ACS's top-level professionals. See Rose Kushner, *Alternatives: New Developments in the War on Breast Cancer* (New York: Warner, 1986).

5. The cancer establishment consists of the American Cancer Society, the National Cancer Institute, and many other comprehensive cancer centers, such as the Dana Farber and the Sloan-Kettering Cancer Center.

6. Samuel S. Epstein, *The Politics of Cancer* (San Francisco: Sierra Club, 1978).

7. American Cancer Society, *Who We Are What We Do Where We're Going* (Atlanta: American Cancer Society, 1983).

8. There are many reasons the cancer establishment became the focus of intense criticism. Readers who are interested in the details of this debate can turn to the excellent works of Samuel Epstein and Ralph Moss, who are the vanguard of the anti-cancer establishment. Samuel S. Epstein, *The Politics of Cancer* (San Francisco: Sierra Club, 1978), Ralph W. Moss, *The Cancer Industry: Unraveling the Politics* (New York: Paragon House, 1989).

9. James T. Patterson, *The Dread Disease: Cancer and Modern American Culture* (Cambridge: Harvard University Press, 1987).

10. Ibid, 244.

11. Ibid, 247.

12. Ibid, 249.

13. Ibid, 232.

14. Jane E. Brody, "Inquiries Soaring on Breast Cancer," *New York Times* (October 1, 1974): 21; Nancy Hicks, "Lesson on Examining Breasts Draws Crowd," *New York Times* (October 19, 1974): 32; Rose Kushner, *Alternatives: New Developments in the War on Breast Cancer* (New York: Warner, 1986).

15. *New York Times*, "Betty Ford Tossing a Football" (October 6, 1974).

16. James T. Patterson, *The Dread Disease: Cancer and Modern American Culture* (Cambridge: Harvard University Press, 1987), 258.

17. Rose Kushner was diagnosed with breast cancer around the same time as Ford and Rockefeller. Kushner subsequently published several books about her experience as a breast cancer patient, and she is best known for

having contributed to education about the Halsted radical mastectomy and its eventual abolishment. Further, she was instrumental in changing the standard practice of doing a breast biopsy and, if malignant tissue was found, proceeding directly to a mastectomy—all the while the woman was under general anesthesia. Therefore, a woman undergoing breast surgery was uncertain about whether she would wake up with one breast or two. Foremost through Kushner's activities, the NCI eventually recommended that a breast biopsy be performed and then in a separate second step, further breast surgery would be performed only if necessary and only after the woman was informed.

18. Kushner covers the circumstances under which the surgeries of Betty Ford and Happy Rockefeller were performed in much detail. A "Halsted radical mastectomy" or a "standard radical" entails the removal of the breast as well as the pectoral muscles of the chest wall and the axillary lymph nodes. Today, if a woman has a mastectomy, she most commonly has a "modified radical mastectomy," which means that breast tissue and most of the axillary lymph nodes are removed, but the pectoral muscles are left intact. See Kushner, *Alternatives*. However, it is also important to note that no surgeon can guarantee a 100 percent removal of the breast tissue when performing a mastectomy. This is an important point to consider for women who now decide to get preventative mastectomies because they are at high risk for developing breast cancer.

19. Carcinoma is a malignant tumor that arises in the epithelium, the tissue that lines the external and internal organs of the body (e.g., breast, lung, stomach, colon, and uterus.) "In situ" refers to the stage of cancer. Staging of cancer is done to determine the presence and site of metastases from a primary tumor in order to plan treatment. Usually the stages are 1 through 4. In situ refers to an abnormal cell growth that has not yet reached Stage 1.

20. Rose Kushner. *Alternatives: New Developments in the War on Breast Cancer* (New York: Warner, 1986), 384f.

21. Byllye Y. Avery. "Breathing Life into Ourselves: The Evolution of the National Black Women's Health Project," *The Black Women's Health Book: Speaking for Ourselves*, edited by Evelyn C. White (Seattle: Seal Press, 1990), 4–10; Judy Norsigian, "The Women's Health Movement in the United States," *WGNRR (Women's Global Network on Reproductive Rights)* 39 (1992) 9–12; Sheryl Burt Ruzek, *The Women's Health Movement: Feminist Alternatives to Medical Control* (New York: Praeger, 1978); Mark K. Zimmerman. "The Women's Health Movement: A Critique of Medical Enterprise and the Position of Women," in *Analyzing Gender: A Handbook of Social Science Research*, edited by Myra Marx Ferree and Beth B. Hess (Newbury Park, Calif.: Sage, 1987), 442–72.

22. Judy Norsigian and Jane Pincus, "Organizing for Change: U.S.A.," in *The New Our Bodies, Ourselves: A Book by and for Women, updated and expanded version for the 1990s*, edited by the Boston Women's Health Book Collective (New York: Touchstone, 1992).

23. Susan Ferraro, "The Anguished Politics of Breast Cancer," *New York Times Magazine* (August 15, 1993):24–27, 58–62; Rose Kushner, *Alternatives: New Developments in the War on Breast Cancer* (New York: Warner, 1986).

24. NABCO's founders were: Rose Kushner, a representative of the Breast Cancer Advisory Center; Diane Blum of Cancer Care, Inc.; Nancy Brinker of the Susan G. Komen Foundation; and Ruth Spear, a patient and author living in New York. Kushner left NABCO when it did not take the political direction she had envisioned and instead decided to take on Congress by founding a political action group called "Breastpak." It dissolved after Kushner's death in 1990. Roberta Altman, *Waking Up/Fighting Back: The Politics of Breast Cancer* (Boston, Mass.: Little Brown & Company, 1996).

25. I label the time period starting roughly with 1990 the post–AIDS era. By "post–AIDS," I mean to characterize that AIDS' organizational response has reached beyond emergence. Many of the AIDS service organizations are firmly in place and funded, and AIDS has firmly established itself as a recognized international health crisis. Since my main focus is not the organizational history of AIDS, I provide the reader merely with a short, overgeneralized history of cancer and AIDS.

26. National Alliance of Breast Cancer Organizations (NABCO) Pamphlet, 1993.

27. Audre Lorde, *The Cancer Journals* (San Francisco: Aunt Lute, 1980).

28. "Silence = Death" came to symbolize AIDS activism and became a well-known icon. Nancy E. Stoller, "Racial Prescriptions for Sexual Permissions: Ideological Messages in AIDS Prevention Materials," Paper presented at *Annual Meeting of the American Sociological Association*, August 19–23 (1995b Washington, D.C.).

29. In chapter 2, I explain in detail the advantages of limiting this study to women activists.

30. Mirko D. Grmek, *History of AIDS: Emergence and Origin of a Modern Pandemic* (Princeton: Princeton University Press, 1990), 183.

31. Dennis Altman, *AIDS in the Mind of America* (Garden City: Anchor Press, 1986); Philip M. Kayal, *Bearing Witness: Gay Men's Health Crisis and the Politics of AIDS* (Boulder; San Francisco; Oxford: Westview Press, 1993); Cindy Patton, *Inventing AIDS* (New York and London: Routledge, 1990); Randy M. Shilts, *And the Band Played On: Politics, People and the AIDS Epidemic* (New York: St. Martin's Press, 1987).

32. Cindy Patton, *Inventing AIDS* (New York and London: Routledge, 1990); Randy M. Shilts, *And the Band Played On: Politics, People and the AIDS Epidemic* (New York: St. Martin's Press, 1987).

33. Cindy Patton, *Inventing AIDS* (New York and London: Routledge, 1990).

34. Cindy Patton, *Inventing AIDS* (New York and London: Routledge, 1990), p. 14; Dennis Altman, *AIDS in the Mind of America* (Garden City: Anchor Press, 1986), Ch. 5.

35. Dennis Altman, *AIDS in the Mind of America* (Garden City: Anchor Press, 1986) and Randy M. Shilts, *And the Band Played On: Politics, People and the AIDS Epidemic* (New York: St. Martin's Press, 1987). Both Dennis Altman and Randy Shilts refer many times to the ACS as the model. For instance,

Shilts writes on p. 122: " . . . but the gay community didn't have time to dawdle in despair. . . . They needed some kind of foundation, like the American Cancer Society or something, that could get warnings out to gay men and pressure the government for more research funds."

36. Dennis Altman, *AIDS in the Mind of America* (Garden City: Anchor Press, 1986), 94.

37. There are many criticisms of Shilts' chronicle of the AIDS crisis. Nevertheless, And the Band Played On became the popular history of the epidemic due to its accessible journalistic style and its adaptation into a TV movie version. On the other hand, Shilts' book is also very controversial within the gay and lesbian community. He has often been criticized for his internalized homophobia that surfaced through his portrayal of "Patient Zero," about a gay man and a foreigner more or less blamed for transmitting HIV. Kevin Cathcart, "Soon To Be Made-For-TV Movie: Randy Shilts, And the Band Played On," *Radical America* 21 (1988): 49–57. Cindy Patton criticizes Shilts for ignoring the structural and historical formation of the gay community that causes his time frame to be at odds with hers and Dennis Altman's, even though all three authors cover the same period. Judy Macks and Caitlin Ryan, "Lesbians Working in AIDS: An Overview of Our History and Experience," in *The Sourcebook on Lesbian/Gay Health Care*, edited by Michael Shernoff and William A. Scott (Washington, D.C.: National Lesbian/Gay Health Foundation, 1988), criticize Shilts' omission of the contribution lesbians made to countering the AIDS epidemic. The early contribution of lesbian women is better covered in Altman's book, published prior to Shilts', and in Patton's works. Shilts' writing is generally insensitive to women's issues and adopts the standpoint of a gay white man as being superior to everyone else. The following quote partially demonstrates this bias; "Jaffe [a CDC official] wondered whether the experts had heard that, away from the comfortable laboratories of the NCI, people were actually dying of this thing [AIDS]. Such a process [the NCI's process] might be all right for delving into the problems of breast cancer or melanoma." Randy M. Shilts, *And the Band Played On: Politics, People and the AIDs Epidemic* (New York: St. Martin's Press, 1987), 82.

38. Judy Macks and Caitlin Ryan, "Lesbians Working in AIDS: An Overview of Our History and Experience," in *The Sourcebook on Lesbian/Gay Health Care*, edited by Michael Shernoff and William A. Scott (Washington, D.C.: National Lesbian/Gay Health Foundation, 1988), 200.

39. Patton's work is important in understanding AIDS activism and organizational responses but has its limitations in that her focus is predominantly on the gay and lesbian community. Cindy Patton, *Inventing AIDS* (New York and London: Routledge, 1990).

40. This describes an overall trend. Of course, it is difficult to date such distinctions exactly and to state them accurately on a national basis. The AIDS epidemic was also differently developed in various parts of the country. Moreover, it has been reported that gay community-based AIDS service organizations, example the Gay Men's Health Crisis (GMHC) in New York City,

estimated that in the early 1980s, 40 percent of its clientele was non-gay. This situation was also created by the fact that gay community-based organizations existed earlier than other organizations, and often non-gays had no other organizations to go to. Dennis Altman *AIDS in the Mind of America* (Garden City: Anchor Press, 1986), 90.

41. Beth E. Schneider "AIDS and Class, Gender, and Race Relations," in *The Social Context of AIDS*, edited by Joan Huber and Beth E. Schneider (Newbury Park, Calif.: Sage, 1992), 35.

42. ACT UP/NY Women and AIDS Book Group, *Women, AIDS, and Activism* (Boston, Mass.: South End Press, 1990); Gena Corea, *The Invisible Epidemic: The Story of Women and AIDS* (New York: HarperCollins, 1992); Carol Leigh, "Further Violations of Our Rights," in *AIDS: Cultural Analysis, Cultural Activism*, edited by Douglas Crimp (Cambridge, Mass.: MIT Press, 1988), 177–81; Gloria Lockett, "Black Prostitutes and AIDS," in *The Black Women's Health Book: Speaking for Ourselves*, edited by Evelyn C. White (Seattle: Seal Press, 1990), 189–92.

43. People with AIDS/ARC, "The Denver Principles," in *Women, AIDS & Activism*, edited by the ACT UP/NY Women and AIDS Book Group (Boston: South End, 1990), 239ff.

44. George M. Carter, *ACT UP, the AIDS War & Activism* (Westfield, N.J.: Open Media, 1992).

45. ACT UP/NY Woman and AIDS Book Group, *Women, AIDS, & Activism* (Boston, Mass.: South End Press, 1990). Gena Corea, *The Invisible Epidemic: The Story of Women and AIDS* (New York: HarperCollins, 1992); Terri Ford, "Women Lead Renewed Uprising," *Women Alive* (winter 1995): 4.

46. Sharon Batt, *Patient No More: The Politics of Breast Cancer* Charlottetown, Canada: gynergy books, 1994); Masha Gessen, "Lesbians and Breast Cancer," in *Advocate* (February 9, 1993); Lisa M. Krieger, "Breast Cancer Activists Look to AIDS Forces," in *San Francisco* (May 5, 1991): A1 and A16; *Examiner*; Alisa Solomon, "The Politics of Breast Cancer," in *Village Voice* (May 14, 1991): 22–27.

47. There is evidence that breast cancer activism draws on both and combines feminist strategies and cultural forms with a disease focus. The disease focus is one of the aspects that breast cancer activists have taken from AIDS organizing. The women's health movement was organized broadly around women's health issues; with AIDS, however, the focus has been narrowed to the immediate concerns about a specific disease instead of broad demands and empowerment messages about women's health or gay and lesbian health.

48. The AIDS "buddy system" refers to a program that many AIDS service organizations have put into place. A "buddy" is a trained person who is assigned to individuals with HIV or AIDS. Depending on need, the buddy does anything from spending time together to going to the movies, cooking, cleaning, shopping, and performing other daily tasks with or for the person with HIV/AIDS.

49. Alisa Solomon, "The Politics of Breast Cancer," in *Village Voice* (May 14, 1991): 22–27.

50. National Coalition of Feminist and Lesbian Cancer Projects, *Technical Assistance Manual for Developing Feminist/Lesbian Cancer Projects* (Washington, D.C.: Mary-Helen-Mautner Project for Lesbians with Cancer and the National Coalition of Feminist and Lesbian Cancer Projects, 1995).

51. Susan M. Love with Karen Lindsey, *Dr. Susan Love's Breast Book* (Reading, Mass.: Addison-Wesley, 1995).

52. The Women's Community Cancer Project in Cambridge, Massachusetts, is an example of such an organization. This organization has actually been credited for pioneering the breast cancer movement's agenda in the direction of linking cancer to the environment. Compare its fact sheets on cancer and the environment and its fact sheet on the American Cancer Society. Sharon Batt, *Patient No More: The Politics of Breast Cancer* (Charlottetown, Canada: Gynergy books, 1994).

53. Michael Castleman, "Breast Cancer Cover Up," *Mother Jones* (May/June 1994): 34, Greenpeace Report and Joe Thornton, *Chlorine, Human Health and the Environment: The Breast Cancer Warning* (Washington, D.C.: Greenpeace, 1993); Women's Environment & Development Organization and Greenpeace, "We Are Rachel's Children, in *Breast Cancer Action* (newsletter, 1994), 4.

54. Women and AIDS Coalition, "Women and AIDS Coalition 1993 Mission and Priorities," in *The Guide to Resources on Women and AIDS*, edited by the Center for Women Policy Studies (Washington, D.C.: Center for Women Policy Studies, 1992), 3f.

55. Ciindy Patton, *Inventing AIDS* (New York and London: Routledge, 1990).

56. Cindy Patton, *Inventing AIDS* (New York and London: Routledge, 1990), 18ff; Urvashi Vaid, *Virtual Equality: The Mainstreaming of Gay and Lesbian Liberation* (New York: Anchor Books, 1995).

57. Cindy Patton, *Inventing AIDS* (New York and London: Routledge, 1990); Urvashi Vaid, *Virtual Equality: The Mainstreaming of Gay and Lesbian Liberation* (New York: Anchor Books, 1995).

58. Wayne Hoffman, "Putting the Gay Back into Gay Men," *Bay Windows* (April 25, 1996): 3, 22; Eric Rofes, *Reviving the Tribe: Regenerating Gay Men's Sexuality and Culture in the Ongoing Epidemic* (New York: Harrington Park Press, 1995); Eric E. Rofes, "Gay Groups vs. AIDS Groups: Averting Civil War in the 1990s," *OUT/LOOK* 2 (1990): 8–17.

CHAPTER 2

1. American Cancer Society, *Cancer Facts & Figures—1996* (Atlanta, Ga.: American Cancer Society, 1996); Catherine C. Boring, Teresa S. Squires, and Tony Tong, *Cancer Statistics 1993* (Atlanta, Ga.: American Cancer Society, 1993).

2. American Cancer Society, "Breast Cancer Facts and Figures, 1997," 1997; (American Cancer Society, "Cancer Facts and Figures 1999," 1999a; American Cancer Society, "Research Shows Different Tumor Characteristics," ACS website: http://www2.cancer.org/zine/001/001_02031999_0.html, 1999b; Susan M. Love with Karen Lindsey, *Dr. Susan Love's Breast Book* (Reading, Mass.: Addison-Wesley, 1995).

3. American Cancer Society, "Breast Cancer Facts and Figures, 1997," 1997; American Cancer Society, "Research Shows Different Tumor Characteristics," ACS website: http://www2.cancer.org/zine/001/001_02031999_0.html, 1999b; Lynn A. Ries, Barry A. Gloeckler, Benjamin F. Miller, Carol L. Hankey, Angela Harras Kosary, and Brenda K. Edwards (eds.), *SEER Cancer Statistics Review, 1973–1991: Tables and Graphs* (Bethesda, Md.: National Cancer Institute, 1994).

4. American Cancer Society, "Breast Cancer Facts and Figures, 1997," 1997; National Cancer Institute, National Institutes of Health, "Cancer Facts: Racial Differences in Breast Cancer Survival," 1994.

5. Jean Hardistry and Ellen Leopold, "Cancer and Poverty: Double Jeopardy for Women," in *Confronting Cancer, Constructing Change: New Perspectives on Women and Cancer*, edited by Midge Stocker (Chicago, Ill.: Third Side Press, 1993).

6. American Cancer Society, *Cancer Facts & Figures—1995* (Atlanta: American Cancer Society, 1995); American Cancer Society, "Research Shows Different Tumor Characteristics," ACS website: http://www2.cancer.org/zine/ 001/001_02031999_0.html, 1999b.

7. National Cancer Institute, National Institutes of Health, "Cancer Facts: Racial Differences in Breast Cancer Survival," 1994.

8. Susan M. Love with Karen Lindsey, *Dr. Susan Love's Breast Book* (Reading, Mass.: Addison-Wesley, 1995).

9. Jean Peterson and Mary Bricker-Jenkins state that Haynes based her analysis on data collected by the National Lesbian Health Care Survey. Judith Bradford and Caitlin Ryan, *The National Lesbian Health Care Survey* (Washington, D.C.: National Lesbian and Gay Health Foundation, 1988); K. Jean Peterson and Mary Bricker Jenkins, "Lesbians and the Health Care System," *Journal of Gay and Lesbian Social Services* 5 no. 1: (1996) 33–47. The National Lesbian Health Care Survey collected data on almost 2,000 lesbians, N = 1925. The sample is, however, not representative of the lesbian population of the United States. Judith Bradford and Caitlin Ryan, *The National Lesbian Health Care Survey* (Washington, D.C.: National Lesbian and Gay Health Foundation, 1988).

10. Ethan E. Bickelhaupt "Alcoholism and Drug Abuse in Gay and Lesbian Persons: A Review of Incidence Studies," *Journal of Gay and Lesbian Social Services* 2 no. 1 (1995) Judith Bradford and Caitlin Ryan, *The National Lesbian Health Care Survey* (Washington, D.C.: National Lesbian and Gay Health Foundation, 1988); Joanne M. Hall, "Alcoholism in Lesbians: Developmental, Symbolic Interactionist, and Critical Perspectives," *Health Care for Women International* 11 no. 1 (1990): 89–107; Katherine A. O'Hanlan, "Lesbians in Health

Research," in *Recruitment and Retention of Women in Clinical Studies*, edited by U.S. Department of Health and Human Services, NIH Publication No. 95-3756, 1995, 101–04; Susan E. Trippet and Joyce Bain, "Physical Health Problems and Concerns of Lesbians," *Women and Health* 20 no. 2 (1993): 59–70.

11. Institute of Medicine, Committee on Lesbian Health Research Priorities, *Lesbian Health: Current Assessment and Directions for the Future* (Washington, D.C.: National Academy Press, 1999).

12. Ibid, 2f.

13. Centers for Disease Control and Prevention, 1998. *HIV/AIDS Surveillance Report*, 1998.

14. National Institute of Allergy and Infectious Diseases, National Institutes of Health, *HIV/AIDS Statistics, NIAID Fact Sheet* (Bethesda, Md.: NIAID/NIH, 1999).

15. National Institute of Allergy and Infectious Diseases, National Institutes of Health, *Women and HIV, NIAID Fact Sheet* (Bethesda, Md.: NIAID/NIH, 1997).

16. Ibid.

17. Centers for Disease Control and Prevention, *HIV/AIDS Surveillance Report*, 1998.

18. Ibid.

19. National Institute of Allergy and Infectious Diseases, National Institutes of Health, *Women and HIV, NIAID Fact Sheet* (Bethesda, Md.: NIAID/NIH, 1997).

20. Centers for Disease Control and Prevention, *HIV/AIDS Surveillance Report*, 1998.

21. Ibid.

22. Rebecca M. Young, *HIV/AIDS and Women Who Have Sex with Women*, presentation to the Institute of Medicine Workshop on Lesbian Health Research Priorities, Georgetown University Conference Center, Washington, D.C., October 6–7, 1997. The current study is funded by the NIDA, entitled, "HIV Risk among Women IDUs Who Have Sex with Women" conducted by Marysol Asencio, Patricia Case, Michael Catts, Sam Friedman, and Amber Hollibaugh.

23. Gena Corea, *The Invisible Epidemic: The Story of Women and AIDs* (New York: HarperCollins, 1992); National Institute of Allergy and Infectious Diseases, National Institutes of Health, *Women and HIV, NIAID Fact Sheet*. Bethesda, Md.: NIAID/NIH, 1997; Sue V. Rosser, *Women's Health—Missing from U.S. Medicine* (Bloomington and Indianapolis: Indiana University Press, 1994).

24. Institute of Medicine, Susan Thaul and Dana Hotra (eds.), *An Assessment of the NIH Women's Health Initiative* (Washington, D.C.: National Academy Press, 1993); Katherine A. O'Hanlan, "Lesbians in Health Research," in *Recruitment and Retention of Women in Clinical Studies*, edited by U.S. Department of Health and Human Services, NIH Publication No. 95-3756, 1995, 101–04; Sue V. Rosser, *Women's Health—Missing from U.S. Medicine*. (Bloomington and Indianapolis: Indiana University Press, 1994); Debbie Ward, "Women and Health Care," in *Women's Health Care: A Comprehensive Handbook*, edited by

Catherine Ingram Fogel and Nancy Fugate Woods (Thousand Oaks, Calif.: Sage, 1995), 111–24.

25. Doug McAdam, "Gender as a Mediator of the Activist Experience: The Case of Freedom Summer," *American Journal of Sociology* 97 March (1992): 1211–40. On pp. 1211ff, Doug McAdam also lists a number of studies that have found various explanations for activism, such as prior contact with a member of the movement, integration into activist networks, and so forth.

26. This perspective has been heavily influenced by the personal comments of William A. Gamson. In addition, he expressed similar thoughts in his presidential address to the Eastern Sociological Society, in which he compared the movements against U.S. military intervention in both Vietnam and El Salvador. Regarding the comparison of these two movements that did not take place simultaneously, he said, "Every collective action process started at a radically different point in the two situations. But if one believes, as I do, that there are certain generic processes present even in two movements as different as these, the challenge is to find lessons that hold across such varying contexts. My particular concern in this essay is with the kind of processes that contribute to long term commitment and solidarity among movement participants. I believe that we can learn from both of these cases about the construction of a 'movement' collective identity and about the quality of social relationships and risk-sharing that contribute to commitment and solidarity." William A. Gamson, "Democratic Participation in Social Movements," in *Presidential Address to the Eastern Sociological Association*, 1990. This presidential address was published later as William A. Gamson "Commitment and Agency in Social Movements," *Sociological Forum* 6 no. 1:27–50.

27. All of the following studies refer to AIDS volunteers: S. M. Chambre, "Volunteers as Witnesses: The Mobilization of AIDS Volunteers in New York City, 1981–1988, *Social Service Review* (1991), 531–47; Philip M. Kayal, *Bearing Witness: Gay Men's Health Crisis and the Politics of AIDS* (Boulder; San Francisco; Oxford: Westview Press, 1993); Halina Maslanka, "Women Volunteers at GMHC," *Women and AIDS: Psychological Perspectives*, edited by Corinne Squire (London & Newbury Park, Calif.: Sage, 1993), 110–25; Allen M. Omoto and A. Lauren Crain, "AIDS Volunteerism: Lesbian and Gay Community-Based Responses to HIV," in *AIDS, Identity, and Community: The HIV Epidemic and Lesbians and Gay Men*, edited by Gregory M. Herek and Beverly Greene (Thousand Oaks, Calif.: Sage, 1995), 187–209; Allen M. Omoto and Mark Snyder, "Basic Research in Action: Volunteerism and Society's Response to AIDS," in *Personality and Social Psychology Bulletin* 16 no. 1 (1990): 162–65; Allen M. Omoto, Mark Snyder, and James P. Berghuis, "The Psychology of Volunteerism: A Conceptual Analysis and a Program of Action Research," in *The Social Psychology of HIV Infection*, edited by J. B. Pryor and G. D. Reeder (Hillsdale, N.J.: Lawrence Erlbaum Associates, 1993), 333–56; Jonathan D. Poullard and Anthony R. D'Augelli, "AIDS Fear and Homophobia Among Volunteers in an AIDS Prevention Program," *Journal for Rural Community Psychology* 10 no. 1 (1989): 29–39; Mark Snyder and Allen M. Omoto, "Volunteerism and Society's

Response to the HIV Epidemic," *Current Directions in Psychological Science* 3 no. 4 (1992): 113–16.

28. Many examples prove that providing services for members of one's community is a political act. For instance, the women's movement created houses for battered women and rape crisis centers that are essentially political service-providing organizations.

29. Wendy Kaminer, *Women Volunteering: The Pleasure, Pain, and Politics of Unpaid Work from 1830 to the Present* (Garden City: Anchor Press, Doubleday & Co. Inc., 1984), 14.

30. Ibid, 4.

31. Ibid.

32. According to Kaminer, a 1981 Gallup poll found that people most likely to volunteer are educated, suburban or rural, upper-income white women who are employed part time. Second, upper-income women who are not the chief wage earners in their family are more likely to volunteer regularly. Wendy Kaminer, *Women Volunteering: The Pleasure, Pain, and Politics of Unpaid Work from 1830 to the Present* (Garden City: Anchor Press, Doubleday & Co. Inc., 1984).

33. This is not to say that working-class women and/or women of color are never volunteers. They, of course, volunteer as well. But whether they volunteer in an organized way that makes them accessible to others or whether they embrace the term *volunteer* for themselves is questionable. For instance, Kaminer writes, "Paid working women, minority women, and women who see themselves as radicals or at least, reformers working to change the system are apt to call themselves community organizers or activists." Wendy Kaminer, *Women Volunteering: The Pleasure, Pain, and Politics of Unpaid Work from 1830 to the Present* (Garden City: Anchor Press, Doubleday & Co. Inc., 1984), 18.

34. Jackie Winnow, "The Politics of Cancer," in *Confronting Cancer, Constructing Change: New Perspectives on Women and Cancer*, edited by Midge Stocker (Chicago, Ill.: Third Side Press, 1993), 153.

35. Cindy Patton writes, "I use the idea of an AIDS service industry— which I understand roughly as the private-sector non-profit organizations devoted exclusively to AIDS work." Cindy Patton, *Inventing AIDS* (New York and London: Routledge, 1990), 13.

36. Breast cancer activism became professionalized through the creation of paid positions, most frequently the position of an executive director. Examples are the National Breast Cancer Coalition, the Mary-Helen-Mautner Project for Lesbians with Cancer, and the Massachusetts Breast Cancer Coalition.

37. Many researchers approach a topic by focusing on leaders in organizations or movements. See, for instance, Barbara Ryan, *Feminism and the Women's Movement: Dynamics of Change in Social Movement, Ideology and Activism* (New York: Routledge, 1992) and Nancy Whittier, *Feminist Generations: The Persistence of the Radical Women's Movement* (Philadelphia: Temple University Press, 1995). For my purposes, this is the wrong approach because it silences certain women, for example women who are HIV-positive. Second, my focus on

understanding organizational culture and how collective identity becomes defined has required that I investigate the boundaries of culture and collective identity.

38. For further details, see the Appendix.

39. As I indicated in the Appendix, I interviewed a total of seventeen women of color.

40. Wendy Kaminer, *Women Volunteering: The Pleasure, Pain, and Politics of Unpaid Work from 1830 to the Present* (Garden City: Anchor Press, Doubleday & Co. Inc., 1984), 18.

41. Susan Liroff, "Challenging the Establishment," in *One in Three: Women with Cancer Confront an Epidemic*, edited by Judith Brady (Pittsburgh and San Francisco: Cleis Press, 1991), 262f.

42. Alisa Solomon, "The Politics of Breast Cancer" in *Village Voice* (May 14, 1991): 27.

43. To simplify the selection of my sample, I made no effort to include bisexual women.

44. Sarah Schulman, *My American History: Lesbian and Gay Life during the Reagan/Bush Years* (New York: Routledge, 1994), 238.

45. On a book tour for her anthology *Dyke Life: From Growing Up to Growing Old*, (New York: Basic Books, 1995). Karla Jay pointed out that the recent feminist book on menopause, *Silent Passage*, by Gail Sheehy (New York: Random House, 1992), neglects to mention lesbians—thereby falsely suggesting that the experience of menopause affects lesbians identically.

46. Roberta Altman, *Waking Up/Fighting Back: The Politics of Breast Cancer* Boston, Mass.: Little Brown & Company, 1996); Barbara Anderson, (ed.), *Women with Cancer: Psychological Perspectives* (New York: Springer Verlag, 1986); Peggy Boyd, *The Silent Wound: A Startling Report on Breast Cancer and Sexuality* (Reading, Mass.: Addison-Wesley, 1984); Lesley Fallowfield with Andrew Clark, *Breast Cancer* (New York: Tavistock/Routledge, 1991); Mimi Greenberg, *Invisible Scars: A Guide to Coping with the Emotional Impact of Breast Cancer* (New York: Walker and Company, 1988). While I was not researching questions of breast reconstruction and so forth, it was pointed out to me by a lesbian breast cancer activist that she has never met a lesbian who chose breast reconstruction after mastectomy.

CHAPTER 3

1. ACT UP/NY Women and AIDS Book Group, *Women, AIDS, and Activism* (Boston, Mass.: South End Press, 1990), 243.

2. I mean by "less well-known celebrities" that we do not know of any women who are HIV-positive or who have AIDS and have been persons with high profiles in their own right, such as Rock Hudson, Robert Mapplethorpe, and many more.

3. Valerie Sacks, "Women and AIDS: An Analysis of Media Misrepresentations," *Social Science and Medicine* 42 no. 1 (1996): 67.

4. Evelynn Hammonds, "Missing Persons: African American Women, AIDS and the History of Disease," *Radical America* 24 no. 2 (1992): 11.

5. Chris Norwood argues this point. She writes: "What is most striking is the lack of coverage of the now extensive efforts of HIV-positive women themselves to contribute to AIDS care and prevention in their communities." Chris Norwood, "Media Coverage on Women and AIDS: Bias, Negative Imagery, and Exclusion of Women's Experts and Sources," in *The Guide to Resources on Women and AIDS*, edited by Center for Women Policy Studies (Washington, D.C.: Center for Women Policy Studies, 1990), 15.

6. Ibid, 5.

7. In the mid-1970s, a number of well-known women went public with their cancer diagnoses. The media reported on these prominent women who underwent breast cancer surgery: "Marvella Bayh, wife of Indiana Senator Birch Bayh, the actress Shirley Temple Black, and [within a month of each other in 1974] Betty Ford and Happy Rockefeller," James T. Patterson, *The Dread Disease: Cancer and Modern American Culture* (Cambridge: Harvard University Press, 1987). This early wave was followed by a number of women who published their accounts about breast cancer, including Betty Rollin, Rose Kushner, Deena Metzger, and Audre Lorde; Rose Kushner *Breast Cancer: A Personal History* (New York: Harcourt Brace, 1975); Rose Kushner, *Why Me? What Every Woman Should Know* (New York: New American Library, 1977); Rose Kushner, *Alternatives: New Developments in the War on Breast Cancer* (New York: Warner, 1986); Audre Lorde, *The Cancer Journals* (San Francisco: Aunt Lute, 1980); Audre Lorde, "Living with Cancer," in *The Black Women's Health Book: Speaking for Ourselves*, edited by Evelyn C. White (Seattle: Seal Press, 1990), 27–37; Deena Metzger, *The Woman Who Slept with Men to Take the War Out of Them* (Culver City, Calif.: Peace Press, 1981); Betty Rollin, *First You Cry* (New York: New American Library, 1976).

8. Susan Ferraro, "The Anguished Politics of Breast Cancer," in *New York Times Magazine* (August 15, 1993): 24–27. The article marked a turning point for various reasons. The picture of a woman with a mastectomy, Matuschka, accompanied by the caption, "You can't look away anymore" on the front cover of the *New York Times Magazine*, provoked a lot of attention beyond the readers of the *New York Times*. The article was reprinted in hundreds of newspapers across the country and dozens around the world, and it was talked about on many news stations. Among breast cancer activists, Matuschka is a controversial figure. She describes herself as an artist and activist and is a member of the New York group WHAM (Women's Health Action and Mobilization). She reminisces over the publication of the *New York Times* article and the printing of her picture on the cover as "the one major advance this culture may have made" in 1993. Matuschka's, "Venus di Milo Has a Problem," *Sappho's Isle* 6, no. 10 (1993): 6, 11. Matuschka's 1993 cover photo was nominated for

the Pulitzer Prize and has generally been received as an example of radical art that changed the way in which people look at breast cancer. Further, the "photo was seen by two million people and garnered more mail than any other cover in the magazine's history. The comments ran from disgruntled cancer survivors who said, 'I feel my privacy has been invaded!' to delighted cancer survivors who said, 'I feel as if a burden has been lifted!' " Delaynie Rudner, "The Censored Scar," in *Gauntlet* 2 no. 9 (1995): 21. See also Rudner's article for a more detailed description of predecessors to Matuschka's mastectomy photo and Breast Cancer Action's difficulties surrounding their breast cancer photo exhibit "Healing Legacies," which was scheduled to be displayed in the United States House of Representative's Cannon Office Building Rotunda in Washington, D.C.

9. Susan Ferraro, "The Anguished Politics of Breast Cancer," in *New York Times Magazine* (August 15, 1993): 25f.

10. Ibid, 58.

11. Within the cancer movement, some of the women without cancer are also active for the first time.

12. I am not looking at cancer from a medical perspective, therefore, I will not talk at all about differences in treatment options and cancer diagnoses. Each cancer diagnosis is different and depends on a variety of factors that belong in the realm of medicine. Therefore, even women with the same type of cancer might have vastly different opportunities to become active because of their health status. Activism means, in a very practical sense, traveling to and from meetings and sitting in meeting rooms for several hours. These are possible physical limitations for women who are not well. Further, there are also differences in life expectancy rates between different types of cancer. These differences deprive women who have a more aggressive or a less treatable type of cancer from participating.

13. Of course, there are also many physical obstacles for HIV-positive women to be active and to participate in a group. As I indicated for women with cancer, the women with HIV have to travel, sit in meetings, and so forth. Because HIV-positive women have a weakened immune system, their involvement and activism might expose them to other factors like sneezing, coughing, and viral illnesses, with which many so-called healthy, HIV-negative people walk around with every day.

14. The segments of the population that are afflicted with cancer or HIV have been discussed in chapter 2.

15. Nevertheless, the women described their HIV-positive results as such a crucial moment in their lives that it caused them to change their lives for the better. I will discuss this point in more detail in the context of motivation.

16. See the creation of the butch–femme roles and survival skills of butches and femmes, Elizabeth Lapovsky Kennedy, and Madeleine Davis, " 'They Was No One to Mess With' ": The Construction of the Butch Role in the Lesbian Community of the 1940s and 1950s," in *The Persistent Desire: A Femme-Butch Reader*, edited by Joan Nestle (Boston, Mass.: Alyson, 1992), 62–

79; Joan Nestle, *A Restricted Country* (Ithaca, N.Y.: Firebrand Books, 1987); Joan Nestle, (ed.), *The Persistent Desire: A Femme–Butch Reader* (Boston, Mass.: Alyson, 1992); See Lillian Faderman, *Odd Girls and Twilight Lovers: A History of Lesbian Life in Twentieth Century America* (New York: Penguin 1991) and Jonathan Katz, *Gay American History: Lesbians and Gay Men in the U.S.A.* (New York: Avon Books, 1976) about both the economic necessity and the increased freedom to which these passing women aspired. Data on women substance abusers show that more than 90 percent of these women experienced sexual abuse as children. One interviewee who works with women substance abusers stated that in her agency substance abuse in women who have been abused as children is close to 100 percent "We are speculating that that may have had something to do with their becoming substance abusers as a way to deal with the pain and all of that that's involved" [AIDS movement]. About the relationship between HIV and sexual abuse in women, see also Gena Corea, *The Invisible Epidemic: The Story of Women and AIDS* (New York: HarperCollins, 1992).

17. Here I refer to a vast variety of programs, some of which are taking place within prisons. One example of such empowerment programs is the following offered in June 1995 by Women of Action, a group that had been formed in 1994 by Boston's AIDS Action Committee's First Women and HIV Advocacy Institute. The pamphlet describing the upcoming "Women and HIV Advocacy Training" included the following statements: "Women of Action is looking for women to join in the effort to influence the legislative/advocacy process. . . . The training is open to women from all communities and backgrounds who are living with HIV and/or do AIDS work in their community. *We encourage participation by women who are HIV-positive*" [emphasis in original]. The program continues: "The training is free of charge. HIV+ women will receive a stipend for their participation in this day of training. Child care and transportation will be paid for upon request."

18. For instance, the NBCC advertisement for Project Lead mentions that committed activists gathered for rigorous training—fourteen-hour days studying highly technical science material. In the future, these workshops will be designed to incorporate on-line communication between teachers and students.

19. Participation in these programs is free, however, one must have the time and money to pay for room and board.

20. The term *resources* is taken from the resource mobilization literature, which also defines what resources are. Barbara Ryan explains: "A resource mobilization framework focuses on the ways a movement creates interest and support for its goals. Resources refer to assets such as money, expertise, media attention, power and votes; however, the primary resource is the people around which the movement is organized." Barbara Ryan, *Feminism and the Women's Movement: Dynamics of Change in Social Movement, Ideology and Activism* (New York: Routledge, 1992), 3. I am not claiming to extend these already existing definitions. My term *personal resources* is micro-oriented.

21. I include nationality and ethnic origin in this list because, within the context of researching AIDS and breast cancer, it was continuously brought to my attention that health and one's relationship to health are first culturally determined. Women who are illegal immigrants have restricted access to health care and are unlikely candidates to become active within either of the two health-related movements.

22. Dennis Altman, *AIDS in the Mind of America* (Garden City: Anchor Press, 1986); Randy M. Shilts, *And the Band Played On: Politics, People and the AIDS Epidemic* (New York: St. Martin's Press, 1987).

23. Michelangelo Signorile, *Queer in America: Sex, the Media, and the Closets of Power* (New York: Random House, 1993).

24. American Cancer Society, "Cancer Facts and Figures 1999," 1999a; Celia Byrne, "Risk Factors: Breast," in *Cancer Rates and Risks*, edited by the National Institutes of Health and the National Cancer Institute, 4th ed. online publication, 1996).

25. National Institute of Allergy and Infectious Diseases, National Institutes of Health, *Women and HIV, NIAID Fact Sheet* (Bethesda, Md.: NIAID/ NIH, 1997).

26. I can only speculate on the numeric distribution, since I have not collected data that represent the entire population of women cancer activists.

27. M. K. Anglin, "Working From the Inside Out: Implications of Breast Cancer Activism for Biomedical Policies and Practices," in *Social Science & Medicine* 44 no. 9 (1997): 1403–15.

CHAPTER 4

1. "Self-interest," as I use it, has to be distinguished from another notion, the "personal," to which I refer in this section as well. The difference is that self-interest refers to being motivated by a gain for oneself; the gain is the goal of one's activism. Being motivated by a personal connection refers to a means of involvement without implying a gain for oneself as the end of activism. My working definition is used against the backdrop of a larger body of literature that uses and defines self-interest theoretically in much more detail than I incorporate here. See also Note 3.

2. "Solidarity" is another term that is widely discussed and theoretically defined in the social movement literature. As I indicated earlier for other terms, such as "self-interest" and the "personal," I can only provide readers with brief working definitions and not theoretical essays on the different usage of these terms.

3. Within social movement literature, self-interest as a motivation for action is often discussed within the rational choice frame. While resource mobilization theory argues that movement participants act as rational actors who make organized decisions to further their interests, Mancur Olson (1965) argues against this line of reasoning. He points out that self-interest is not

enough of a motivation, since a rational actor could be riding free on the efforts of others and still perceive collective goods. This argument has often been criticized since it shortchanges rational behavior to individual profit maximization. For this discussion in the literature, see Myra Marx Ferree, "The Political Context of Rationality: Rational Choice Theory and Resource Mobilization," in *Frontiers in Social Movement Theory*, edited by Aldon Morris and Carol McClurg Mueller (New Haven, Ct.: Yale University Press, 1992), 29–52; Mancur Olson, *The Logic of Collective Action* (Cambridge, Mass.: Harvard University Press, 1965).

4. See the section "Gay Men and Cancer Activists"

5. Anthony Giddens, *Modernity and Self-Identity* (Stanford: Stanford University Press, 1991), 99.

6. Until the CDC revised its definition of AIDS for the third time in 1993, women's symptoms of AIDS had not been included. The new definition included invasive cervical cancer, pulmonary tuberculosis, and recurrent pneumonia to the case definition list. Carol Glassman, "Lesbians and HIV Disease," *Journal of Gay and Lesbian Social Services* 2 no. 3–4 (1995): 61–74. Some maintained their criticism of an androcentric definition of AIDS, because the most common signs of a compromised immune system in women, such as severe, persistent vaginal candidiasis, pelvic inflammatory disease, human papillomavirus, genital herpes, cervical dysplasia, and molluscum contagiosum, have not been included in the definition. Glassman, ibid.; Patricia E. Stevens, "Lesbians and HIV: Clinical Research, and Policy Issues," *American Journal of Orthopsychiatry* 63 no. 2 (1993): 289–94.

7. Chris Norwood, "Alarming Rise in Deaths," *MS.* 17 no. 1 (1988): 65, 67.

8. National Institute of Allergy and Infectious Diseases, National Institutes of Health, *Women and HIV, NIAID Fact Sheet* (Bethesda, Md.: NIAID/NIH, 1997); B. Schable, S. Y. Chu, and T. Diaz, "Characteristics of Women 50 Years of Age or Older with Heterosexually Acquired AIDS," *American Journal of Public Health* 86 no. 11 (1996): 1616–18; K. Siegel, D. Karus, and V. H. Raveis, "Testing and Treatment Behaviour of HIV-Infected Women: White, African-American, Puerto Rican Comparisons, *AIDS Care* 9 No. 3 (1997): 297–309.

9. The serum HIV-antibody test has been available since 1985.

10. The NIH states that in mammography among forty- to forty-nine-year-olds, up to one-fourth of all breast cancers will be missed, and 10 percent will be missed in fifty- to sixty-nine-year-old women. NIH Consensus Statement, 1997 Jan. 21–23, "Breast Cancer Screening for Women Ages 40–49" 15 (January 21–23, 1997) Bethesda, Md.

11. American Cancer Society, "Breast Cancer Facts and Figures, 1997," 1997.

12. The so-called cancer establishment is, according to Ralph W. Moss, "distinct circles of power . . . which, while differing among themselves on many issues, are sufficiently cohesive and interlocking to form a 'cancer establishment.' This establishment effectively controls the shape and the direction of cancer prevention, diagnosis, and therapy in the United States." Ralph W.

Moss, *The Cancer Industry: Unraveling the Politics* (New York: Paragon House, 1989), 389. Further, he explains, "Within the cancer field it appears that the major decisions are made at the tops of four or five organizations. . . . At the pinnacles of power, the scientists and physicians are often subordinated to the control of laypersons. . . . More often than not, these laypersons are the very people with the greatest vested interest in the outcome of the cancer problem." Moss, ibid, 390. The four most powerful organizations, according to Moss, that have a business interest in favoring the cure of cancer over its prevention are the Memorial Sloan-Kettering Cancer Center, the American Cancer Society, the National Cancer Institute, and the Food and Drug Administration. Moss, ibid.

13. According to statistics from the American Cancer Society, the specificity of mammography allows for 10 percent of false positives and false negatives in 6 percent to 24 percent of cases. American Cancer Society, "Breast Cancer Facts and Figures, 1997," 1997. The National Women's Health Network breaks down the sensitivity by age groups. Their fact sheet states, "In women over fifty, a single mammogram misses 13% of the cancer actually present (a false negative result). Each year, 2% of the women who have mammograms will be told that their mammograms indicate problems when they do not have cancer (a false positive result). For women under fifty, the accuracy of mammography is much worse. The false positive rate is 3% and the false negative rate is a startling 38%. In other words, if mammography were given to every woman in her forties who had breast cancer that was too small to feel, nearly 40 out of 100 cancers would be missed." National Women's Health Network, "Mammography in Women under 50" (Washington, D.C.: National Women's Health Network, updated).

14. Chris Norwood, "Media Coverage on Women and AIDS: Bias, Negative Imagery, and Exclusion of Women's Experts and Sources," in *The Guide to Resources on Women and AIDS*, edited by the Center for Women Policy Studies (Washington, D.C.: Center for Women Policy Studies, 1990), 16.

15. Among the accounts of women with cancer, one can find examples of women who describe how their doctors have not listened to their health complaints. See Cindy Winslow, "A Letter to My Doctor," in *One in Three: Women with Cancer Confront an Epidemic*, edited by Judith Brady (Pittsburgh and San Francisco, Cleis Press, 1991), 129–36.

16. Sandra Butler and Barbara Rosenblum, *Cancer in Two Voices* San Francisco: Spinsters, 1991), i.

17. Ibid, 41.

18. Ibid, 73.

19. Hence, malpractice suits or lawsuits are one instrument that can be used for social change as it has been done in the context of many other movements. There have been lawsuits within the civil rights movement, environmental pollution is often subject to demand judicial repercussions, and other politically motivated court battles the right to same-sex marriage, for instance, and so forth.

20. Here it is important to recall that within cancer activism one can also find women who are without the disease but who are new to political activism as well. On the other hand, one can also find politically experienced women who were diagnosed with cancer.

21. One of the specific communities that has been mentioned by HIV-positive first-time activists is the IV-drug-using community. While the women activists might target the women substance abusers, I am sure that they will also hand out "works" to men. In this sense, the communities to which the HIV activists are referring are not included when one talks broadly about women.

22. The National Cancer Institute points to the following risk factors: (1) age: the risk of breast cancer increases as a woman gets older; (2) family history: the risk of getting cancer increases if a woman's female blood relatives had the disease—a hereditary explanation; (3) late childbirth: a woman's risk for breast cancer increases if she has never given live birth or if she had her first full-term pregnancy after age thirty. Further risk factors that researchers found increased the occurrence of breast cancer included menstruation at an early age (before twelve) or menopause at a late age (after fifty-five). The risk also increased with eating a high-fat diet, being overweight, or having a high consumption of alcohol. National Institutes of Health and National Cancer Institute, *What You Need to Know About Breast Cancer* (National Cancer Institute, Bethesda, Md., 1993). In spite of these risk factors, the reality is that 75 percent to 80 percent of all diagnosed breast cancers are in women who have none of these risk factors. Karen Lindsey, "Breast Cancer: Who's at Risk?" *Sojourner* (September 1989); National Institutes of Health and National Cancer Institute, ibid. "Approximately 80% of all cancers are in some way related to environmental factors," according to even the most conservative scientists. Rita Arditti and Tatiana Schreiber, "Breast Cancer: The Environmental Connection," *Resist* no. 246 (1992): 1–8. Nevertheless, the debate about what causes cancer is ongoing, and researchers take different stands.

23. Patricia Hill Collins, *Black Feminist Thought: Knowledge, Consciousness, and the Politics of Empowerment* (New York; London: Routledge, 1991), 129.

24. Ibid, 132.

25. Patricia Hill Collins refers to bell hooks' essay "toward a revolutionary feminist pedagogy" in bell hooks, *Talking Back: Thinking Feminist, Thinking Black* (London: Sheba Feminist Publishers, 1989).

26. Patricia Hill Collins, *Black Feminist Thought: Knowledge, Consciousness, and the Politics of Empowerment* (New York; London: Routledge, 1991), 131f.

27. As with other groups, lesbians are also found as examples of other types. I mentioned lesbians among the motivational type, diagnosis. Some lesbians are first-time activists, and others identify with communities of color; still others choose a broader political approach.

28. Melissa A. McNeill, "Who Are "We"?: Exploring Lesbian Involvement in AIDS Work," (Northampton, Mass.: Smith College School for Social Work, Thesis, 1991).

29. Nancy Stoller, "Lesbian Involvement in the AIDS Epidemic: Changing Roles and Generational Differences," in *Women Resisting AIDS: Feminist Strategies of Empowerment*, edited by Beth E. Schneider and Nancy E. Stoller (Philadelphia: Temple University Press, 1995a), 270–85.

30. Ibid, 275.

31. Her critique was originally published as an interview in 1987. See Cynthia Yockey, "AIDS: Sidetracking Feminism. A Conversation with Sonia Johnson," *Lambda Rising Book Report* 1 no. 2 (1987):1, 5. This interview is the basis for a chapter in Johnson's book, which was published in 1989. See Sonia Johnson, *Wildfire: Igniting the She/Volution* (Albuquerque: Wildlife Books, 1989). The chapter is entitled, "Gay Rights and AIDS: Men's Issues Sidetracking Feminism again."

32. Sonia Johnson, *Wildlife: Igniting the She/Volution* (Albuquerque: Wildfire Books, 1989), 187f.

33. Generally, George Weinberg is accredited with being the first to present the concept of homophobia. G. Weinberg, *Society and the Healthy Homosexual* (Boston: Alyson, 1972).

34. I am in no position to decide whether solidarity with gay men, essentially what I call a gay and lesbian community focus, has existed alongside a feminist community focus. For instance, Stoller seems to argue that the feminist motivation was secondary. Even though she uses different language, her title "Equal rights for women/lesbians within the AIDS world" best summarizes what I call motivation due to feminist consciousness. She defines her perspective as follows: "Soon after women became engaged in the work of the epidemic, a second perspective began to be expressed: that women, as AIDS workers and as people at risk for AIDS, were the victims of sexism and secondary status." Nancy Stoller, "Lesbian Involvement in the AIDS Epidemic: Changing Roles and Generational Differences," in *Women Resisting AIDS: Feminist Strategies of Empowerment*, edited by Beth E. Schneider and Nancy E. Stoller (Philadelphia: Temple University Press, 1995a), 278. In contrast, reading Gena Corea, who focuses entirely on women and the AIDS crisis, makes it plausible that straight women and lesbians became involved in AIDS work on behalf of women right away. See Gena Corea *The Invisible Epidemic: The Story of Women and AIDS* (New York: HarperCollins, 1992).

35. Judith B. Cohen "HIV Risk among Women Who Have Sex with Women," *San Francisco Epidemiologic Bulletin* no. 4 (1993): 26.

36. On the other hand, lesbian self-identity does not predict behavior, since self-identified lesbians may have sex with men. Judith B. Cohen, "HIV Risk among Women Who Have Sex with Women," *San Francisco Epidemiologic Bulletin* 9 no. 4 (1993): 25–30; Rebecca Cole and Sally Cooper, "Lesbian Exclusion from HIV/AIDS Education: Ten Years of Low Risk Identity and High Risk Behavior," *Siecus Report* (Dec./Jan. 1991): 18–23; Carol Glassman, "Lesbians and HIV Disease," *Journal of Gay and Lesbian Social Services* 2 no. 3–4 (1995): 61–74. Institute of Medicine, Committee on Lesbian Health Research Priori-

ties. 1999. *Lesbian Health, Current Assessment and Directions for the Future*. Washington, D.C.: National Academy Press.

37. Gena Corea, *The Invisible Epidemic: The Story of Women and AIDS* (New York: HarperCollins, 1992), 20.

38. Carol Glassman, "Lesbians and HIV Disease," *Journal of Gay and Lesbian Social Services* 2 no. 3–4 (1995): 61–74.

39. This is an overgeneralization. There are HIV-positive lesbians, however, who usually have a different political background. There are few exceptional early cases of HIV-positive lesbians who have been active within AIDS, Liz Wolfe. Again, there are no reliable data available on the serostatus of the lesbian community, and I have no quantitative data on women AIDS activists at a national level.

40. Jackie Winnow, "Lesbians Evolving Health Care: Our Lives Depend On It," in *Cancer as a Women's Issue: Scratching the Surface* edited by Midge Stocker (Chicago, Ill.: Third Side Press, 1991), 23–35.

41. Ibid, 23.

42. Ibid.

43. I make this statement without national data on the age distribution of lesbian cancer activists and lesbian AIDS activists. I think, however, that it is safe to exclude age as a factor behind lesbians' involvement in AIDS or cancer activism. My reasoning for doing so is that one would have to take into account the lesbian AIDS activists who were in the AIDS movement in the early 1980s but left later on because of "burnout." The inclusion of these early activists would even out the assumed age gap between AIDS and breast cancer activists.

44. At the end of her article, Susan Shapiro calls for a meeting to discuss plans for a Women's Community Cancer Project. This meeting took place and marked the founding of the Women's Community Cancer Project (WCCP) in Cambridge, Massachusetts. A few years later, in 1991, some women left the WCCP and founded the Massachusetts Breast Cancer Coalition (MBCC).

45. Susan Shapiro, "Cancer As a Feminist Issue," *Sojourner* (September 1989).

46. Examples of these frames that appeal to women who share the same political frames are the various fact sheets that cancer organizations publish. For instance, the WCCP in Cambridge, Massachusetts, published a number of fact sheets on different cancers. The most dominant underlying message was to highlight the environmental connection to various cancers. As discussed later, other frames are also possible, for example, anti-racism and cancer, which appeals to communities of color; homophobia and cancer, which appeals to gays and lesbians; fact sheets on access; and so on.

47. I assume that women who have solely spiritual concerns will much more likely be found within the service and caretaking arenas of AIDS organizations, which are the aspects of organizational AIDS responses that I excluded from my sample.

48. The women to whom I am referring here are HIV-positive women whom I encountered and with whom I had preliminary talks. I considered them as interviewees. The interviews never took place because the women were not part of AIDS activism. The women told me that they wanted to but that they felt estranged from the existing groups due to their different class and racial backgrounds. They felt that groups made up of men who matched their race and class backgrounds were their only option. They disliked this option because they preferred to be with a majority of women.

49. I make no claims that my sample of interviewees is representative, however, I find it noteworthy and more than coincidental that I did not encounter any straight white middle-class women at all. This is not to say that they do not exist among AIDS activists. I see this more as a trend that those who are activists are a minority segment among women AIDS activists. Further, my guess is that straight white middle-class women are much easier to find in the other segments of organizational responses to AIDS, such as the helping positions and service professions. Omoto and Crain researched AIDS volunteerism in 1990–1991 in AIDS organizations that focus on care and assistance for people with HIV. One of their findings is that the gay volunteers are predominantly male (84 percent to 16 percent female), whereas this distribution is reversed among the non-gay volunteers (82 percent straight women to 18 percent straight men). See Allen M. Omoto and A. Lauren Crain, "AIDS Volunteerism: Lesbian and Gay Community-Based Responses to HIV," in AIDS, Identity, and Community: The HIV Epidemic and Lesbians and Gay Men, edited by Gregory M. Herek and Beverly Greene (Thousand Oaks, Calif.: Sage, 1995), 187–209.

50. Dennis Altman, AIDS in the Mind of America. (Garden City: Anchor Press, 1986); Philip M. Kayal, Bearing Witness: Gay Men's Health Crisis and the Politics of AIDS (Boulder; San Francisco; Oxford: Westview Press, 1993); Cindy Patton, Inventing AIDS (New York and London: Routledge, 1990); Randy M. Shilts, And the Band Played On: Politics, People and the AIDS Epidemic (New York: St. Martin's Press, 1987).

51. Dennis Altman, AIDS in the Mind of America (Garden City: Anchor Press, 1986); Beth E. Schneider, "AIDS and Class, Gender, and Race Relations," in The Social Context of AIDS, edited by Joan Huber and Beth E. Schneider (Newbury Park, Calif.: Sage, 1992).

52. ACT UP/NY Women and AIDS Book Group, Women, AIDS, and Activism (Boston, Mass.: South End Press, 1990); Gena Corea, The Invisible Epidemic: The Story of Women and AIDS (New York: HarperCollins, 1992); Carol Leigh, "Further Violations of Our Rights," in AIDS: Cultural Analysis, Cultural Activism, edited by Douglas Crimp (Cambridge, Mass.: MIT Press, 1988), 177–81; Gloria Lockett, "Black Prostitutes and AIDS," in The Black Women's Health Book: Speaking for Ourselves, edited by Evelyn C. White (Seattle: Seal Press, 1990), 189–92.

53. People with AIDS/ARC, "The Denver Principles," in Women, AIDS & Activism, edited by the ACT UP/NY Women and AIDS Book Group (Boston: South End, 1990), 239ff.

54. These issues or collective identities are discussed in greater detail in chapters 5 and 6, which focus on the various collective identities of AIDS and cancer activism.

55. Judy Brady is a well-known figure within breast cancer activism. She is also the editor of an anthology. See Judith Brady, *One in Three: Women with Cancer Confront an Epidemic* (Pittsburgh and San Francisco: Cleis Press, 1991).

CHAPTER 5

1. William A. Gamson, "Commitment and Agency in Social Movements," *Sociological Forum* 6 no. 1 (1991): 27–50.

2. Ibid, 41.

3. Nancy Whittier, *Feminist Generations: The Persistence of the Radical Women's Movement* (Philadelphia: Temple University Press, 1995), 15.

4. Throughout the text, I have made the point that the cancer movement emerged based on a feminist analysis of cancer.

5. Whereas within the AIDS movement, gender has to be negotiated differently because male and female activists are involved in it.

6. The concept of positivist feminism is used as a feminist critique of science. Positivist feminism was the first phase of criticizing science, which still exists, but it is often, from today's point of view, not a very radical approach. See Janet Saltzman Chafetz, "Some Thoughts By an Unrepentant 'Positivist' Who Considers Herself a Feminist Nevertheless," presented at the *Annual Meeting of the American Sociological Association* (August 1990) as a prime example. Sometimes this type of feminism is also called "add [women] on and stir" or feminist empiricism. A critique of feminist empiricism, which is the same as positivist feminism, has been put forward by the so-called standpoint theorists. Standpoint theorists start thinking from women's lives and question the assumption of an objective reality that underlies positivist feminism. See Sandra Harding, *Whose Science? Whose Knowledge? Thinking From Women's Lives* (Ithaca, N.Y.: Cornell University Press, 1991). Harding also offers a detailed critique of feminist empiricism.

7. From the press release of the NBCC (National Breast Cancer Coalition) in 1991. This notion of inclusivity also holds true on the first level of collective identity, the organizational level:

The WCCP (Women's Community Cancer Project) demands: "[I]increase[d] funding, *through new allocations*, for research on cancers of the female reproductive organs . . . to whatever level is necessary to allow for *meaningful* research in *decreased incidence and decreased mortality among women of all races, ethnic groups and social classes*" [emphasis in original]. Note that sexual orientation is not included here. Women's Community Cancer Project, "Demands to the NCI and the U.S. Government," in *Confronting Cancer, Constructing Change: New Perspectives on Women and Cancer*, edited by Midge Stocker (Chicago, Ill.: Third Side Press, 1993), 261–63.

The MBCC (Massachusetts Breast Cancer Coalition) demands "Improved access for *all* women to screening" [emphasis added].

8. See chapter 2.

9. To claim inclusivity of women with all types of cancers and to operate with this false equality of different types of cancer also minimizes the differences in survival times, the different medical knowledge in treating one cancer versus another, the difference in screening tools for various cancers, or even the existing limited knowledge about the causes of certain cancers.

10. A useful essay making the connection between invisibilizing women and the gender neutrality of organizations in the working world is Joan Acker, "Hierarchies, Jobs, Bodies: A Theory of Gendered Organizations," *The Social Construction of Gender*, edited by Judith Lorber and Susan A. Farrell (Newbury Park, Calif.: Sage, 1991), 162–79, who also touches on issues of sexuality.

11. "Gender, or what I would call 'heterogenders,' is the asymmetrical stratification of the sexes in relation to the historically varying institutions of patriarchal heterosexuality. Reframing gender as heterogender foregrounds the relation between heterosexuality and gender. . . . As a materialist feminist concept, heterogender de-naturalizes the 'sexual' as the starting point for understanding heterosexuality and connects institutionalized heterosexuality with the gender division of labor and the patriarchal relations of production." Chrys Ingraham, "The Heterosexual Imaginary: Feminist Sociology and Theories of Gender," *Sociological Theory* 12 no. 2 (1994): 204.

12. The most prominent critic has been Adrienne Rich, in her well-known essay "Compulsory Heterosexuality and Lesbian Existence." Adrienne Rich, "Compulsory Heterosexuality and Lesbian Existence," in *Powers of Desire: The Politics of Sexuality*, edited by Ann Snitow, Christine Stansell, and Sharon Thompson (New York: Monthly Review Press, 1983), 177–205. She discusses the heterosexual bias of feminist and women's health books. Rich writes: *"Our Bodies, Ourselves,* the Boston Women's Health Collective's best-seller . . . devotes a separate (and inadequate) chapter to lesbians . . . whose message is that heterosexuality is most women's life preference." Rich, ibid, 202.

13. See chapter 4.

14. This point is problematic, since no reliable statistics are available on the lesbian community and the prevalence of HIV and breast cancer in this special population. The common understanding is that lesbians are more prone to developing breast cancer than contracting HIV. Estimates of this sort also depend largely on one's definition of a lesbian.

15. Earlier I discussed the risk and incidence of breast cancer. Most respondents have disregarded the findings of Suzanne Haynes's report that estimated the risk of breast cancer in lesbians at 1 in 3. The majority of respondents doubted this statistic, since it was derived from nongeneralizable data on the lesbian community.

16. Adrienne Rich, "Compulsory Heterosexuality and Lesbian Existence," in *Powers of Desire: The Politics of Sexuality*, edited by Ann Snitow, Christine Stansell, and Sharon Thompson (New York: Monthly Review Press, 1983), 178.

17. George A. Appleby, "AIDS and Homophobia/Heterosexism." *Journal of Gay and Lesbian Social Services* 2 no. 3–4 (1995): 1–23; Warren J. Blumenfeld, (ed.), *Homophobia: How We All Pay the Price* (Boston: Beacon Press, 1992); Warren J. Blumenfeld and Diane Raymond, *Looking at Gay and Lesbian Life* (Boston: Beacon Press, 1993).

18. While I define gay culture here as an environment in which being gay or lesbian is normative, I discuss later the gender dynamics of the culture.

19. As indicated for gay culture, "gay positive" refers to an environment that treats various sexual orientations as equal, although this does not mean that equality encompasses gender equality as well.

20. Elizabeth V. Spelman, *Inessential Woman: Problems of Exclusion in Feminist Thought* (Boston: Beacon Press, 1988), 182.

21. George A. Appleby, "AIDS and Homophobia/Heterosexism," *Journal of Gay and Lesbian Social Services* 2 no. 3–4 (1995): 1–23; Warren J. Blumenfeld, (ed.), *Homophobia: How We All Pay the Price* (Boston: Beacon Press, 1992); Warren J. Blumenfeld and Diane Raymond, *Looking at Gay and Lesbian Life* (Boston: Beacon Press, 1993).

22. For this point, it is important to know how my own sexual orientation affected the interview situation. I did not present myself prior to an interview as a lesbian. I also did nothing to disguise my sexual identity. This generally caused the situation where lesbian interviewees knew about my sexual orientation because they are experienced in "reading sexuality." My experience with straight women showed far more variability. Two straight women asked me about my sexual orientation after or during the interview, and I told them. The majority of straight respondents, however, gave no indication of how they perceived me with regard to my sexual orientation. I had different readings of the silences. I divided straight women into two categories. One entailed the majority who are not interested in questioning or knowing someone else's sexual orientation. There are, of course, a variety of possible reasons for that. Within the other category of straight women, I detected subtle differences in behavior, demeanor, and so forth. Even though these women did not ask me about my sexual orientation, I assumed that they knew, at least by the end of the interview due to two possible reasons for that. First, the straight women might have just learned to "read" who is a lesbian and who is not. Second, for some straight women, questions about sexual orientation, as raised during the interview, are an indication that I am a lesbian. These women operate on the assumption that non-lesbians would not have asked these questions.

23. Bette S. Tallen, "How Inclusive Is Feminist Theory? Questions for Lesbians?" in *Lesbian Philosophies and Cultures*, edited by Jeffner Allen (Albany, N.Y.: State University of New York Press, 1990), 254f.

24. This is the same rule that operates in Romance languages, which differentiate between female and male nouns. Feminist linguists decried the power implications of language rules in regard to gender. For instance, in French, as long as one man is in a group of 100 women, one will refer to the

group with the male pronoun because it is the default form. In Spanish, an all-women group, *las amigas*, turns into *los amigos* as soon as one man joins.

25. Julia Penelope, "The Lesbian Perspective," in *Lesbian Philosophies and Cultures*, edited by Jeffner Allen (Albany, N.Y.: State University of New York Press, 1990), 103.

26. The term *lesbian culture* is hotly debated. Some claim that it exists, but others claim that in a male-dominated society (patriarchy) we can hardly talk about women's culture, let alone lesbian culture. The debate is at the core of an essay by Ann Ferguson, "Is There a Lesbian Culture?" in *Lesbian Philosophies and Cultures*, edited by Jeffner Allen (Albany, N.Y.: State University of New York Press, 1990), 63–68.

27. The "sex wars" started around 1981; the Barnard Conference on Sexuality in 1982 is often quoted as their beginning. The "sex wars" refer to an intense time within the women's and the lesbian movement when a divisive battle was fought around issues of sexuality. On one side of the battle line was the anti-pornography group (WAP), led by Andrea Dworkin and others, who violently opposed pornography, butch–femme relationships, sadomasochism, and any other forms of expressive female sexuality. Women who were attacked for being femmes and engaging in certain sexual practices were accused of being anti-feminist, engaging in unequal patriarchal power sex, having a false consciousness, and so forth. For further details about this debate, see Dennis Altman, *AIDS in the Mind of America* (Garden City: Anchor Press, 1986); Joan Nestle, *A Restricted Country* (Ithaca, N.Y.: Firebrand Books, 1987); Barbara Ryan, *Feminism and the Women's Movement: Dynamics of Change in Social Movement, Ideology and Activism* (New York: Routledge, 1992); Ann Snitow, Christine Stansell, and Sharon Thompson (eds.), *Powers of Desire: The Politics of Sexuality* (New York: Monthly Review Press, 1983); Adele M. Stan (ed.), *Debating Sexual Correctness: Pornography, Sexual Harassment, Date Rape, and the Politics of Sexual Equality* (New York: Delta, 1995).

28. Larry Goldsmith, "Ask. Tell." *Resist* (1995) 4 no. 5: 1.

29. Ibid.

CHAPTER 6

1. Sharon R. Kurtz, "All Kinds of Justice: Labor & Identity Politics," Boston College, the Graduate School of Arts and Sciences, Department of Sociology (dissertation), 1994.

2. Ibid, 171.

3. Unfortunately one consequence of singling out sexual orientation from the multitude of collective identities, for example, race, class might reinforce the false assumption that sexual orientation is a white issue, since the previous chapter did not pay any attention to race. Ideally, I would have integrated all different collective identities into one chapter but could not due to the complexity of the material and the arguments.

4. Elizabeth V. Spelman, *Inessential Woman: Problems of Exclusion in Feminist Thought* (Boston: Beacon Press, 1988), 185f.

5. Additive analysis of oppression rests on two key premises: The first is dichotomous "either/or thinking," for example, man/woman, black/white. The second is that these pairs are ranked into a dominant and a subordinate part. Oppression therefore appears quantifiable, as though it were possible to determine that one group is more oppressed than another. See Patricia Hill Collins, "Toward a New Vision: Race, Class, and Gender as Categories of Analysis and Connection," in *Race, Sex & Class* 1 no. 1 (1993): 25–45.

6. Elizabeth V. Spelman, *Inessential Woman: Problems of Exclusion in Feminist Thought* (Boston: Beacon Press, 1988).

7. Naming race and class within the mission statements of cancer organizations is quite frequent. Some examples appear in chapter 5.

8. Here it is important to recall the difference between personal and collective identity, as explained in chapter 5. Membership of straight and lesbian women (personal identity or social location of members) does not lead to a collective identity around sexuality. Therefore, broadening one's constituency through more numeric diversity by having women of color or poor women as members does not in itself constitute a change in the movement's collective identity. See William A. Gamson, "Commitment and Agency in Social Movements," *Sociological Forum* 6 no. 1 (1991): 27–50.

9. Elizabeth V. Spelman, *Inessential Woman: Problems of Exclusion in Feminist Thought* (Boston: Beacon Press, 1988).

10. Barbara Omolade in Elizabeth V. Spelman, *Inessential Woman: Problems of Exclusion in Feminist Throught* (Boston: Beacon Press, 1988), 13.

11. There have been many more examples that proved differences due to a certain racial background. Differences in motivations are discussed in chapter 4, and the perception by women of color that political activism is a white enterprise is discussed in chapter 2.

12. P. M. Beemsterboer, P. G. Warmerdam, R. Boer, and H. J. de Koning, "Radiation Risk of Mammography Related to Benefit in Screening Programmes: A Favourable Balance?" *Journal of Medical Screening* 5 no. 2 (1998): 81–7; S. W. Fletcher, "Breast Cancer Screening among Women in Their Forties: An Overview of the Issues," *Journal of the National Cancer Institute. Monographs:* no. 22 (1997) 5–9; Susan M. Love with Karen Lindsey, *Dr. Susan Love's Breast Book* (Reading, Mass.: Addison-Wesley, 1995).

13. P. M. Beemsterboer, P. G. Warmerdam, R. Boer, and J. H. de Koning, "Radiation Risk of Mammography Related to Benefit in Screening Programmes: A Favourable Balance?" *Journal of Medical Screening* 5 no. 2 (1998): 81–7.

14. M. K. Anglin, "Working From the Inside Out: Implications of Breast Cancer Activism for Biomedical Policies and Practices," *Social Science & Medicine* 44 no. 9 (1997): 1403–15.

15. National Cancer Institute, "Cancer Facts: Screening Mammograms," 1998. While the American Cancer Society and the National Cancer Institute recommend mammography screening of women in their forties, the National

Institutes of Health (NIH) does not make the same recommendation. Instead, the NIH states that every woman in her forties should decide for herself. NIH Consensus Statement, "Breast Cancer Screening for Women Ages 40–49" (January 21–23, 1997) 15: 1–35.

16. By women celebrities, I mean women who are famous in their own right and who are HIV-positive. Within AIDS, this has been the case for men only (e.g., Magic Johnson and Arthur Ashe).

17. Rachel Carson, *Silent Spring* (New York: Houghton Mifflin, 1962).

18. Sandra Steingraber, " 'If I Live to be 90 Still Wanting to Say Something': My Search for Rachel Carson, in *Confronting Cancer, Constructing Change: New Perspectives on Women and Cancer*, edited by Midge Stocker (Chicago, Ill.: Third Side Press, 1993), 181–200. Objectivity had not yet been challenged in the 1960s. Further, in the 1960s, having cancer had a different stigma than in the 1990s; one did not speak about cancer in the 1960s with the same matter-of-fact attitude that one does in the 1990s.

19. "Rachel Carson Was Right" proclaims a button distributed and designed by the Women's Community Cancer Project in Cambridge, Massachusetts. Further, newsletters and other organizations are named after Rachel Carson.

20. Sylvia Dunnavant, *Celebrating Life: African American Women Speak Out About Breast Cancer* (Dallas: USFI, Inc., 1995), 16.

21. Audre Lorde, *The Cancer Journals* (San Francisco: Aunt Lute, 1980).

22. A good example is the annual "Outwrite" conference in Boston. At this gay and lesbian writers' conference, an Audre Lorde lecture has been established. In 1996, Cheryl Clarke, who gave the lecture, paid tribute to Toni Cade Bambara, yet another woman who died of breast cancer. See Cheryl Clarke "Tributes to the Lives and Works of Toni Cade Bambara and Jerri L. Jewell," *Gay Community News* 24 no. 3–4 (1996): 10, 32–33. Many other women come to mind, including Pat Parker, an African-American poet and lesbian. The Gay and Lesbian Community Center in New York named its library in her honor.

23. Lesbian cancer organizations selected Chastity Bono as their spokesperson. She is an out-lesbian who frequently speaks about her loss of a lover to breast cancer. Bono is the daughter of Cher and the late Sonny Bono. While this definitely speaks to the lesbian community, it engages neither communities of color nor changes the perception of the cancer movement as a white middle-class one.

24. There is also a possibility of some overlap between cancer and AIDS. Bill T. Jones choreographed a piece called "Still/Here," which actually spoke generally to any life-threatening illness and explicitly to breast cancer. But whereas the AIDS movement successfully uses such cultural events for fund-raising, for example, the cancer movement hardly ever becomes visible. Another crossover example is Patti LaBelle. At the local level, she was invited to a joint AIDS and breast cancer fund-raising event for the gay and lesbian community-based health center (Fenway) and the Massachusetts Breast Can-

cer Coalition. LaBelle spoke out about both HIV/AIDS and breast cancer, to which she has lost three sisters. Kevin John Lindsay, "Making the Connections," in *Bay Windows* 13 (November 9, 1995): 24.

25. Francis Calpotura and Rinku Sen, "PUEBLO Fights Lead Poisoning," in *Unequal Protection: Environmental Justice and Communities of Color*, edited by Robert D. Bullard (San Francisco: Sierra Club, 1994), 254.

26. In Boston, the ACS established the William B. Price Memorial Unit. Dr. Price was a physician who practiced in the inner city for many years and died of cancer in 1974. The Price unit serves the inner-city, racially mixed, and low-income communities of Boston (including Chinatown, Dorchester, Roxbury, Mattapan, the South End, and Jamaica Plain). In addition to many volunteers, the unit is staffed with one paid part-time and two paid full-time employees. The Price unit specializes in diversity, community connections, and breast health. It provides direct services (e.g., medical services, free wigs, free mammograms) to cancer patients, but it also does education and advocacy in these communities. American Cancer Society, *Dr. William B. Price Memorial Unit Fact Sheet* (Boston, Mass.: American Cancer Society, Greater Boston Regional Center, undated).

27. Nancy E. Stoller, "Racial Prescriptions for Sexual Permissions: Ideological Messages in AIDS Prevention Materials" presented at the *Annual Meeting of the American Sociological Association*, August 19–23 1995 (Washington, D.C.: 1995).

28. Ibid, 3.

29. There was a mainstreaming of AIDS that severed AIDS organizations from their more radical grassroots liberationist roots of the early years. For this point, see Cindy Patton, *Inventing AIDS* (New York and London: Routledge, 1990).

30. Maintaining a stand toward monied interests and ideological messages and staying true to the fight for equal resources for all will be even more important in the future, for two reasons. First, the incidence of HIV or HIV transmission is moving more into the disenfranchised segments of the population (women—especially women of color—and communities of color). If AIDS shifts into these segments, the question arises of whether funding will continue. Second, recent medical-scientific gains have discovered life-prolonging drugs that are very costly. They raise the question of whether someone's economic situation will determine the length of her life in that those who can afford the drugs will live longer and those who cannot will die sooner.

31. Here I am referring not just to the arguments presented in chapters 5 and 6 but also to other arguments presented elsewhere in this book. For instance, in chapter 3, I talked about the challenging advocacy training that requires the educational background that mostly middle-class women have.

32. Robert Gottlieb, *Forcing the Spring: The Transformation of the American Environmental Movement* (Washington, D.C.: Island Press, 1993); Celene Krauss, "Women of Color on the Front Line," in *Unequal Protection: Environmental Justice and Communities of Color*, edited by Robert D. Bullard (San Francisco:

Sierra Club, 1994), 256–71; Paul Mohai, "Public Concern and Elite Involvement in Environmental-Conservation Issues," *Social Science Quarterly* 66 no. 4
(1985): 820–38. The environmental movement is a considerable
overgeneralization. One has to distinguish between the clearly white, conservative, and heavily middle-class wildlife conservationist movement and the
more progressive anti-toxins movement. Often, the anti-toxins movement, to
which the environmental justice movement also belongs, is presented as the
radical wing of the environmental movement.

33. Andrew Szasz argues that the grassroots movement against toxics is
one led by women. Between 70 percent and 80 percent of the leadership of the
local leaders are women. Further, he mentions that women within this movement were encouraged to think about situations in which they felt degraded,
dismissed, patronized, used, or ignored by men. Andrew Szasz, *EcoPopulism:
Toxic Waste and the Movement for Environmental Justice* (Minneapolis: University
of Minnesota Press, 1994).

34. Robert Gottlieb, *Forcing the Spring: The Transformation of the American
Environmental Movement* (Washington, D.C.: Island Press, 1993).

35. Ibid.

36. In chapter 5, I defined "heterosexist" if the feminist analysis is generated from straight women's perspectives. See the new coalitions between cancer and other health organizations and environmental organizations. While
these coalitions highlight ethnic, racial, and class diversity, they hardly ever
include sexual orientation in their demands. See Rachel's Children, newsletter
(June 1995) 1; Rachel's Children: Fighting for Our Lives, *Women Health and the
Environment* (Newsletter, February 1995).

37. Carolyn Merchant, *Earthcare: Women and the Environment* (New York:
Routledge, 1996).

38. Women's Voices for the Earth website.

39. For instance, chapter 5 also addresses the heterosexist culture of the
women's health movement.

40. Barbara Ryan, *Feminism and the Women's Movement: Dynamics of Change
in Social Movement, Ideology and Activism* (New York: Routledge, 1992), 125.

41. I discussed earlier that AIDS activism by women and lesbians has
been criticized from a feminist perspective by claiming that it distracts women
from their own issues. See chapter 4.

42. Barbara Ryan, *Feminism and the Women's Movement: Dynamics of Change
in Social Movement, Ideology and Activism* (New York: Routledge, 1992).

43. The Rainbow Endowment is a nonprofit organization that contributes
funds derived from the use of the Visa Rainbow Card to nonprofit groups that
support programs on lesbian and gay health, culture, and civil rights across
the country. *Rainbow News* 1 (Spring 1996).

44. In 1996, the nonprofit organization Rainbow Endowment distributed
individual donations of $8,500 to the following six groups: AIDS Information
Network, Astrea National Lesbian Action Foundation, Community Research
Initiative on AIDS, *National Breast Cancer Coalition*, National Lesbian and Gay

Health Association, and National Center for Lesbian Rights. [emphasis added]. *Rainbow News* 1 (Fall 1996).

CHAPTER 7

1. Susan Bordo, *Unbearable Weight: Feminism, Western Culture and the Body.* Berkeley: University of California Press, 1993).

2. Ibid, 73.

3. This statement looks merely at the diseases cancer and AIDS. Other than that, it has to be used with caution for the following reasons. First, as Susan Sontag points out in her work, people with cancer were once denied the dignity of being informed about their cancer diagnosis. Second, due to their gender status, women are marked as "other" in a male-dominated society.

4. Exceptions to this rule exist in the context of breast cancer charities. For instance, Lisa Belkin writes that in 1989 Ralph Lauren "teamed up with Katherine Graham, the former publisher of the *Washington Post*, and founded the Nina Hyde Center for Breast Cancer Research at Georgetown University Medical Center. 'I thought I could save her,' Lauren says of Hyde, a longtime fashion editor at the *Post*, who died shortly after the center opened. 'I told Nina I would try my best.' Like countless other people around the country, Lauren was personally touched by the disease, but when wealthy people are touched, amazing things can start to happen. In the years since Hyde's death, Lauren has spent millions of his own dollars and raised millions more to support the center." Lisa Belkin, "How Breast Cancer Became this Year's Hot Charity," in *New York Times Magazine* (December 22, 1996): 44. Another well-known example of a man who became active due to his personal relationship with a woman who died of cancer is Gene Wilder, husband to Gilda Radner.

5. *Chicago Sun-Times*, 1992. "Patients Find Help at US TOO" (July 20, 1992): 14; US TOO, "Organization Introduction," website www.ustoo.com, 1998b.

6. US TOO, "Organization Introduction" website www.ustoo.com, 1998b.

7. Men's Health Network Coalition, website www.menshealthnetwork.org., 1998.

8. National Prostate Cancer Coalition, "About NPCC," website www.4npcc.org., 1998.

9. Men's Health Network Coalition, website www.menshealthnetwork.org., 1998.

10. US TOO, *Hot Sheet* (March 1998).

11. Studies have focused on gender inequality within social movements. McAdam, for example, found significant differences in the meaning that activism has for male and female activists. Doug McAdam, "Gender as a Mediator of the Activist Experience: The Case of Freedom Summer," in *American Journal of Sociology* 97 March (1992): 1211–40.

12. It is always complicated to generalize about lesbians, because data have not been collected.

13. If one were to pursue a macroanalysis, the AIDS and breast cancer movements are differently positioned in the "cycle of protest." Sidney Tarrow defines "cycle of protest" as "a phase of heightened conflict and contention across the social system, which includes: a rapid diffusion of collective action from more mobilized to less mobilized sectors; a quickened pace of innovation in the forms of contention; new or transformed collective action frames; a combination of organized and unorganized participation; and sequences of intensified interaction between challengers and authorities which can end in reform, repression, and sometimes revolution." Sidney Tarrow, *Power in Movement: Social Movements, Collective Action and Politics* (New York: Cambridge University Press, 1994), 153.

14. Here I rely heavily on Nancy Whittier, *Feminist Generations: The Persistence of the Radical Women's Movement* (Philadelphia: Temple University Press, 1995).

15. Ibid.

16. Ibid, 257.

17. See chapter 3 for this discussion.

18. I argued in chapter 3 that some gay men have much in common with first-time cancer activists, in that their first exposure to activism was with AIDS; further, they share the racial and socioeconomic backgrounds with first-time cancer activists.

19. Doug McAdam, "Recruitments to High-Risk Activism: The Case of Freedom Summer," *American Journal of Sociology* 92 no. 1 (1986): 64–90; Doug McAdam, "Micromobilization Context and Recruitment to Activism," in *From Structure to Action: Comparing Movement Participation across Cultures*, edited by Bert Klandermans, Hanspeter Kriesi, and Sydney Tarrow (Greenwich, Ct.: JAI Press, 1988), 125–54.

20. Bert Klandermans and Sydney Tarrow, "Mobilization into Social Movements: Synthesizing European and American Approaches, in *From Structure to Action: Comparing Movement Participation across Cultures*, edited by Bert Klandermans, Hanspeter Kriesi, and Sydney Tarrow (Greenwich, Ct.: JAI Press, 1988), 1–38; David A. Snow, Louis A. Zurcher, and Sheldon Ekland-Olson, "Social Networks and Social Movements: A Microstructural Approach to Differential Recruitment," *American Sociological Review* 45 October (1980): 787–801.

21. I paraphrase Prudence Posner, who writes about James Jennings' work on "The Politics of Black Empowerment": "Community organization in African-American neighborhoods cannot be understood as simply community organization with a black face." Prudence S. Posner, "Introduction," in *Dilemmas of Activism: Class, Community, and the Politics of Local Mobilization*, edited by Joseph M. Kling and Prudence S. Posner (Philadelphia: Temple University Press, 1990), 10.

22. Nancy Whittier, *Feminist Generations: The Persistence of the Radical Women's Movement* (Philadelphia: Temple University Press, 1995), 15.

23. Alberto Melucci quoted in Arlene Stein, "Sisters and Queers: The Decentering of Lesbian Feminism," in *Cultural Politics and Social Movements,* edited by Marcy Darnovsky, Barbara Epstein, and Richard Flacks (Philadelphia: Temple University Press, 1995), 144.

24. My usage of the term *transformative consciousness* is similar to the usage of Kennedy et al. in their essay on transformative populism. Marie Kennedy and Chris Tilly, with Mauricio Gaston, "Transformative Populism and the Development of a Community of Color," in *Dilemmas of Activism: Class, Community, and the Politics of Local Mobilization,* edited by Joseph M. Kling and Prudence S. Posner (Philadelphia: Temple University Press, 1990), 302–24.

25. Ibid, 313.

26. Gloria Anzaldua "La Prieta," in *This Bridge Called My Back: Writings by Radical Women of Color,* edited by Cherrie Moraga and Gloria Anzaldua (Watertown, Mass.: Persephone Press, 1981), 205.

27. Audre Lorde, *Sister Outsider: Essays and Speeches* (Freedom, Calif.: The Crossing Press, 1984), 142.

28. Doug McAdam, "Culture and Social Movements," in *New Social Movements: From Ideology to Identity,* edited by Enrique Larana, Hank Johnston, and Joseph R. Gusfield (Philadelphia: Temple University Press, 1994), 36–57.

29. Wini Breines, *Community and Organization in the New Left: 1962–1968* (South Hadley, Mass.: J. F. Bergin, 1982).

30. June Jordan, quoted in Patricia Hill Collins, "Toward a New Vision: Race, Class, and Gender as Categories of Analysis and Connection," in *Race, Sex & Class* 1 no. 1 (1993): 40.

31. Alberto Melucci, *Nomads of the Present: Social Movements and Individual Needs in Contemporary Society* (Philadelphia: Temple University Press, 1989).

32. Debra Friedman and Doug McAdam, "Collective Identity and Activism: Networks, Choices and the Life of a Social Movement," in *Frontiers in Social Movement Theory,* edited by Aldon Morris and Carol McClurg Mueller (New Haven, Ct.: Yale University Press, 1992), 164.

33. Centers for Disease Control and Prevention, *HIV/AIDS Surveillance Report,* 1998.

34. Ibid.

35. *Cancer Weekly* "Sickness and Politics: The Influence of Disease Advocates: Cancer vs. AIDS, Washington, D.C." (June 8, 1992): 5.

References

Acker, Joan. 1991. "Hierarchies, Jobs, Bodies: A Theory of Gendered Organizations." Pp. 162-79 in *The Social Construction of Gender*, ed. Judith Lorber and Susan A. Farrell. Newbury Park, Calif.: Sage.

ACT UP/NY Women and AIDS Book Group. 1990. *Women, AIDS, and Activism*. Boston, Mass.: South End Press.

Altman, Dennis. 1986. *AIDS in the Mind of America*. Garden City: Anchor Press.

Altman, Roberta. 1996. *Waking Up/Fighting Back: The Politics of Breast Cancer*. Boston, Mass.: Little Brown & Company.

American Cancer Society. 1983. *Who We Are What We Do Where We're Going*. Atlanta: American Cancer Society.

———. 1995. *Cancer Facts & Figures—1995*. Atlanta: American Cancer Society.

———. 1996. *Cancer Facts & Figures—1996*. Atlanta: American Cancer Society.

———. 1997. "Breast Cancer Facts and Figures, 1997."

———. 1999a. "Cancer Facts and Figures 1999."

———. 1999b. "Research Shows Different Tumor Characteristics." ACS website: http://www2.cancer.org/zine/001/001_02031999_0.html.

———. Undated. *Dr. William B. Price Memorial Unit Fact Sheet*. Boston, Mass.: American Cancer Society, Greater Boston Regional Center.

Anderson, Barbara L., ed. 1986. *Women with Cancer: Psychological Perspectives*. New York: Springer Verlag.

Anglin, M. K. 1997. "Working From the Inside Out: Implications of Breast Cancer Activism for Biomedical Policies and Practices." *Social Science & Medicine* 44: 1403–15.

Anzaldua, Gloria. 1981. "La Prieta." Pp. 198–209 in *This Bridge Called My Back: Writings by Radical Women of Color*, ed. Cherrie Moraga and Gloria Anzaldua. Watertown, Mass.: Persephone Press.

Appleby, George A. 1995. "AIDS and Homophobia/Heterosexism." *Journal of Gay and Lesbian Social Services* 2: 1–23.

Arditti, Rita, and Tatiana Schreiber. 1992. "Breast Cancer: The Environmental Connection." *Resist* no. 246: 1–8.

Associated Press. 1993. "Breast Cancer Risk in Lesbians Put at 1 in 3," *Boston Globe* (February 5): 12.

Avery, Byllye Y. 1990. "Breathing Life into Ourselves: The Evolution of the National Black Women's Health Project." Pp. 4–10 in *The Black Women's Health Book: Speaking for Ourselves*, ed. Evelyn C. White. Seattle: Seal Press.

Batt, Sharon. 1994. *Patient No More: The Politics of Breast Cancer*. Charlottetown, Canada: gynergy books.

Beemsterboer, P. M., P. G. Warmerdam, R. Boer, and H. J. de Koning. 1998. "Radiation Risk of Mammography Related to Benefit in Screening Programmes: A Favourable Balance?" *Journal of Medical Screening* 5: 81–7.

Belkin, Lisa. 1996. "How Breast Cancer Became This Year's Hot Charity." *New York Times Magazine*. (December 22): 40, 42–46, 52, 55, 57.

Bickelhaupt, Ethan E. 1995. "Alcoholism and Drug Abuse in Gay and Lesbian Persons: A Review of Incidence Studies." *Journal of Gay and Lesbian Social Services* 2: 5–14.

Blumenfeld, Warren J., ed. 1992. *Homophobia: How We All Pay the Price*. Boston, Mass.: Beacon Press.

Blumenfeld, Warren J., and Diane Raymond. 1993. *Looking at Gay and Lesbian Life*. Boston, Mass.: Beacon Press.

Bordo, Susan. 1993. *Unbearable Weight: Feminism, Western Culture and the Body*. Berkeley: University of California Press.

Boring, Catherine C., Teresa S. Squires, and Tony Tong. 1993. *Cancer Statistics 1993*. Atlanta, Ga.: American Cancer Society.

Boyd, Peggy. 1984. *The Silent Wound: A Startling Report on Breast Cancer and Sexuality*. Reading, Mass.: Addison-Wesley.

Bradford, Judith, and Caitlin Ryan. 1988. *The National Lesbian Health Care Survey*. Washington, D.C.: National Lesbian and Gay Health Foundation.

Brady, Judith, ed. 1991. *One in Three: Women with Cancer Confront an Epidemic*. Pittsburgh and San Francisco: Cleis Press.

Breines, Wini. 1982. *Community and Organization in the New Left: 1962–1968*. South Hadley, Mass.: J. F. Bergin.

Brody, Jane E. 1974. "Inquiries Soaring on Breast Cancer." *New York Times* (October 1): 21.

Butler, Sandra, and Barbara Rosenblum. 1991. *Cancer in Two Voices*. San Francisco: Spinsters.

Byrne, Celia. 1996. "Risk Factors: Breast." In *Cancer Rates and Risks* 4th ed. the National Institutes of Health and the National Cancer Institute; online publication.

Calpotura, Francis, and Rinku Sen. 1994. "PUEBLO Fights Lead Poisoning." Pp. 234–55 in *Unequal Protection: Environmental Justice and Communities of Color*, ed. Robert D. Bullard. San Francisco: Sierra Club.

Cancer Weekly. 1992. "Sickness and Politics: The Influence of Disease Advocates: Cancer vs. AIDS, Washington, D.C." (June 8): p. 5.

Carson, Rachel. 1962. *Silent Spring*. New York: Houghton Mifflin.

Carter, George M. 1992. *ACT UP, the AIDS War & Activism*. Westfield, N.J.: Open Media.

Castleman, Michael. 1994. "Breast Cancer Cover Up." *Mother Jones* (May/June): 34.

Cathcart, Kevin. 1988. "Soon To Be a Made-For-TV Movie: Randy Shilts, And the Band Played On." *Radical America* 21: 49–57.

Centers for Disease Control and Prevention. 1998. *HIV/AIDS Surveillance Report*.

Chafetz, Janet Saltzman. 1990. "Some Thoughts By an Unrepentant 'Positivist' Who Considers Herselof a Feminist Nevertheless." Presented at the *Annual Meeting of the American Sociological Association* (August).

Chambre, Susan M. 1991. "Volunteers As Witnesses: The Mobilization of AIDS Volunteers in New York City, 1981–1988." *Social Service Review* 65: 531–47.

Chicago Sun-Times. 1992. "Patients Find Help at US TOO." (July 20): 14.

Clarke, Cheryl. 1996. "Tributes to the Lives and Works of Toni Cade Bambara and Jerri L. Jewell." *Gay Community News* 24: 10, 32–33.

Cohen, Judith B. 1993. "HIV Risk among Women Who Have Sex with Women." *San Francisco Epidemiologic Bulletin* 9: 25–30.

Cole, Rebecca, and Sally Cooper. 1991."Lesbian Exclusion from HIV/AIDS Education: Ten Years of Low Risk Identity and High Risk Behavior." *Siecus Report* (Dec./Jan.): 18–23.

Collins, Patricia Hill. 1991. *Black Feminist Thought: Knowledge, Consciousness, and the Politics of Empowerment*. New York; London: Routledge.

Collins, Patricia Hill. 1993. "Toward a New Vision: Race, Class, and Gender as Categories of Analysis and Connection." In *Race, Sex & Class* 1: 25–45.

Corea, Gena. 1992. *The Invisible Epidemic: The Story of Women and AIDS*. New York: HarperCollins.

Dunnavant, Sylvia. 1995. *Celebrating Life: African American Women Speak Out About Breast Cancer*. Dallas: USFI, Inc.

Epstein, Samuel S. 1978. *The Politics of Cancer*. San Francisco: Sierra Club.

Faderman, Lillian. 1991. *Odd Girls and Twilight Lovers: A History of Lesbian Life in Twentieth Century America*. New York: Penguin.

Fallowfield, Lesley, with Andrew Clark. 1991. *Breast Cancer*. New York: Tavistock/Routledge.

Ferguson, Ann. 1990. "Is There a Lesbian Culture?" Pp. 63–88 in *Lesbian Philosophies and Cultures*, ed. Jeffner Allen. Albany, N.Y.: State University of New York Press.

Ferraro, Susan. 1993. "The Anguished Politics of Breast Cancer." *New York Times Magazine* (August 15): 24–27, 58–62.

Ferree, Myra Marx. 1992. "The Political Context of Rationality: Rational Choice Theory and Resource Mobilization." Pp. 29–52 in *Frontiers in Social Movement Theory*, ed. Aldon Morris and Carol McClurg Mueller. New Haven, Ct.: Yale University Press.

Fletcher, S. W. 1997. "Breast Cancer Screening among Women in Their Forties: An Overview of the Issues." *Journal of the National Cancer Institute. Monographs* (22): 5–9.

Ford, Terri. 1995. "Women Lead Renewed Uprising." *Women Alive* (winter): 4.

Friedman, Debra, and Doug McAdam. 1992. "Collective Identity and Activism: Network, Choices and the Life of a Social Movement." Pp. 156–73 in *Frontiers in Social Movement Theory*, ed. Aldon Morris and Carol McClurg Mueller. New Haven, Ct.: Yale University Press.

Gamson, William A. 1990. "Democratic Participation in Social Movements." *Presidential Address to the Eastern Sociological Association* (March 24)

———. 1991. "Commitment and Agency in Social Movements." *Sociological Forum* 6: 27–50.

Gessen, Masha. 1993. "Lesbians and Breast Cancer." *Advocate* (February 9): 44–48.

Giddens, Anthony. 1991. *Modernity and Self-Identity*. Stanford: Stanford University Press.

Glassman, Carol. 1995. "Lesbians and HIV Disease." *Journal of Gay and Lesbian Social Services* 2: 61–74.

Goldsmith, Larry. 1995. "Ask. Tell." *Resist* 4: 1–2.

Gottlieb, Robert. 1993. *Forcing the Spring: The Transformation of the American Environmental Movement*. Washington, D.C.: Island Press.

Greenberg, Mimi. 1988. *Invisible Scars: A Guide to Coping with the Emotional Impact of Breast Cancer*. New York: Walker and Company.

Greenpeace Report and Joe Thornton. 1993. *Chlorine, Human Health and the Environment: The Breast Cancer Warning*. Washington, D.C.: Greenpeace.

Grmek, Mirko D. 1990. *History of AIDS: Emergence and Origin of a Modern Pandemic*. Princeton: Princeton University Press.

Hall, Joanne M. 1990. "Alcoholism in Lesbians: Developmental, Symbolic Interactionist, and Critical Perspectives." *Health Care for Women International* 11: 89–107.

Hammonds, Evelynn. 1992. "Missing Persons: African American Women, AIDS and the History of Disease." *Radical America* 24: 7–23.

Harding, Sandra. 1991. *Whose Science? Whose Knowledge?: Thinking From Women's Lives*. Ithaca, N.Y.: Cornell University Press.

Hardisty, Jean, and Ellen Leopold. 1993. "Cancer and Poverty: Double Jeopardy for Women." Pp. 213–30 in *Confronting Cancer, Constructing Change: New Perspectives on Women and Cancer*, ed. Midge Stocker. Chicago, Ill.: Third Side Press.

Hicks, Nancy. 1974. "Lesson on Examining Breasts Draws Crowd." *New York Times* (October 19): 32.

Hoffman, Wayne. 1996. "Putting the Gay Back into Gay Men." *Bay Windows* (April 25): 3, 22.

hooks, bell. 1989. *Talking Back: Thinking Feminist, Thinking Black*. London: Sheba Feminist Publishers.

Ingraham, Crys. 1994. "The Heterosexual Imaginary: Feminist Sociology and Theories of Gender." *Sociological Theory* 12: 203–19.

Institute of Medicine, Committee on Lesbian Health Research Priorities. 1999. *Lesbian Health: Current Assessment and Directions for the Future*. Washington, D.C.: National Academy Press.

Institute of Medicine, Susan Thaul and Dana Hotra, eds. 1993. *An Assessment of the NIH Women's Health Initiative*. Washington, D.C.: National Academy Press.

Johnson, Sonia. 1989. *Wildfire: Igniting the She/Volution*. Albuquerque: Wildfire Books.

Kaminer, Wendy. 1984. *Women Volunteering: The Pleasure, Pain, and Politics of Unpaid Work from 1830 to the Present*. Garden City: Anchor Press, Doubleday & Co. Inc.

Katz, Jonathan. 1976. *Gay American History: Lesbians and Gay Men in the U.S.A.* New York: Avon Books.

Kayal, Philip M. 1993. *Bearing Witness: Gay Men's Health Crisis and the Politics of AIDS*. Boulder; San Francisco; Oxford: Westview Press.

Kennedy, Elizabeth Lapovsky, and Madeline Davis. 1992. " 'They Was No One to Mess With': The Construction of the Butch Role in the Lesbian Community of the 1940s and 1950s." Pp. 62–79 in *The Persistent Desire: A Femme–Butch Reader*, ed. Joan Nestle. Boston, Mass.: Alyson.

Kennedy, Marie, and Chris Tilly, with Mauricio Gaston. 1990. "Transformative Populism and the Development of a Community of Color." Pp. 302–24 in *Dilemmas of Activism: Class, Community, and the Politics of Local Mobilization*, ed. Joseph M. Kling and Prudence S. Posner. Philadelphia: Temple University Press.

Klandermans, Bert, and Sydney Tarrow. 1988. "Mobilization into Social Movements: Synthesizing European and American Approaches." Pp. 1–38 in *From Structure to Action: Comparing Movement Participation across Cultures*, ed. Bert Klandermans, Hanspeter Kriesi, and Sydney Tarrow. Greenwich, Ct.: JAI Press.

Krauss, Celene. 1994. "Women of Color on the Front Line." Pp. 256–71 in *Unequal Protection: Environmental Justice and Communities of Color*, ed. Robert D. Bullard. San Francisco: Sierra Club.

Krieger, Lisa M. 1991. "Breast Cancer Activists Look to AIDS Forces." *San Francisco Examiner*. (May 5): A1 and A16.

Kurtz, Sharon R. 1994. "All Kinds of Justice: Labor & Identity Politics." Boston College, the Graduate School of Arts and Sciences, Department of Sociology (dissertation).

Kushner, Rose. 1975. *Breast Cancer: A Personal History*. New York: Harcourt Brace.
———. 1977. *Why Me? What Every Woman Should Know*. New York: New American Library.
———. 1986. *Alternatives: New Developments in the War on Breast Cancer*. New York: Warner.

Leigh, Carol. 1988. "Further Violations of Our Rights." Pp. 177–81 in *AIDS: Cultural Analysis, Cultural Activism*, ed. Douglas Crimp. Cambridge, Mass.: MIT Press.

Lindsay, Kevin John. 1995. "Making the Connections." *Bay Windows* 13 (November 9): 24.

Lindsey, Karen. 1989. "Breast Cancer: Who's at Risk?" *Sojourner* (September).

Liroff, Susan. 1991. "Challenging the Establishment." Pp. 260–65 in *One in Three: Women with Cancer Confront an Epidemic*, ed. Judith Brady. Pittsburgh; San Francisco: Cleis Press.

Lockett, Gloria. 1990. "Black Prostitutes and AIDS." Pp. 189–92 in *The Black Women's Health Book: Speaking for Ourselves*, ed. Evelyn C. White. Seattle: Seal Press.

Lorde, Audre. 1980. *The Cancer Journals*. San Francisco: Aunt Lute.

———. 1984. *Sister Outsider: Essays and Speeches*. Freedom, Calif.: The Crossing Press.

———. 1990. "Living with Cancer." Pp. 27–37 in *The Black Women's Health Book: Speaking for Ourselves*, ed. Evelyn C. White. Seattle: Seal Press.

Love, Susan M., with Karen Lindsey. 1995. *Dr. Susan Love's Breast Book*. Reading, Mass.: Addison-Wesley.

Macks, Judy, and Caitlin Ryan. 1988. "Lesbians Working in AIDS: An Overview of Our History and Experience." Pp. 198–201 in *The Sourcebook on Lesbian/Gay Health Care*, ed. Michael Shernoff and William A. Scott. Washington, D.C.: National Lesbian/Gay Health Foundation.

Maslanka, Halina. 1993. "Women Volunteers at GMHC." Pp. 110–25 in *Women and AIDS: Psychological Perspectives*, ed. Corinne Squire. London & Newbury Park, Calif.: Sage.

Matuschka. 1993. "Venus di Milo Has a Problem." *Sappho's Isle* 6: 6, 11.

McAdam, Doug. 1986. "Recruitment to High-Risk Activism: The Case of Freedom Summer." *American Journal of Sociology* 92: 64–90.

———. 1988. "Micromobilization Contexts and Recruitment to Activism." Pp. 125–54 in *From Structure to Action: Comparing Movement Participation across Cultures*, ed. Bert Klandermans, Hanspeter Kriesi, and Sydney Tarrow. Greenwich, Ct.: JAI Press.

———. 1992. "Gender as a Mediator of the Activist Experience: The Case of Freedom Summer." *Amercian Journal of Sociology* 97: 1211–40.

———. 1994. "Culture and Social Movements." Pp. 36–57 in *New Social Movements: From Ideology to Identity*, ed. Enrique Larana, Hank Johnston, and Joseph R. Gusfield. Philadelphia: Temple University Press.

McNeill, Melissa A. 1991. "Who Are 'We'?: Exploring Lesbian Involvement in AIDS Work" Northampton, Mass.: Smith College School for Social Work (thesis).

Melucci, Alberto. 1989. *Nomads of the Present: Social Movements and Individual Needs in Contemporary Society*. Philadelphia: Temple University Press.

Men's Health Network Coalition. 1998. Website: www.menshealthnetwork.org.

Merchant, Carolyn. 1996. *Earthcare: Women and the Environment*. New York: Routledge.

Metzger, Deena. 1981. *The Woman Who Slept with Men to Take the War Out of Them*. Culver City, Calif.: Peace Press.

Mohai, Paul. 1985. "Public Concern and Elite Involvement in Environmental-Conservation Issues." *Social Science Quarterly* 66: 820–38.

Moss, Ralph W. 1989. *The Cancer Industry: Unraveling the Politics*. New York: Paragon House.

National Alliance of Breast Cancer Organizationis (NABCO). 1993. Pamphlet.

National Cancer Institute. 1998. "Cancer Facts: Screening Mammograms."

National Cancer Institute, National Institutes of Health. 1994. "Cancer Facts: Racial Differences in Breast Cancer Survival."

National Coalition of Feminist and Lesbian Cancer Projects. 1995. *Technical Assistance Manual for Developing Feminist/Lesbian Cancer Projects*. Washington, D.C.: Mary-Helen-Mautner Project for Lesbians with Cancer and the National Coalition of Feminist and Lesbian Cancer Projects.

National Institute of Allergy and Infectious Diseases, National Institutes of Health. 1997. *Women and HIV, NIAID Fact Sheet*. Bethesda, Md.: NIH.

National Institute of Allergy and Infectious Diseases, National Institutes of Health. 1997. *Women and HIV, NIAID Fact Sheet*. Bethesda, Md.: NIH.

National Institute of Allergy and Infectious Diseases, National Institutes of Health. 1999. *HIV/AIDS Statistics, NIAID Fact Sheet*. Bethesda, Md.: NIH.

National Institutes of Health and National Cancer Institute. 1993. *What You Need to Know About Breast Cancer*. Bethesda, Md.: National Cancer Institute.

National Prostate Cancer Coalition. 1998. "About NPCC." Website: www.4npcc.org.

National Women's Health Network. Undated. "Mammography in Women under 50." Washington, D.C.: National Women's Health Network.

Nestle, Joan. 1987. *A Restricted Country*. Ithaca, N.Y.: Firebrand Books.

———. (ed.). 1992. *The Persistent Desire: A Femme–Butch Reader*. Boston, Mass.: Alyson.

New York Times. 1974. "Betty Ford Tossing a Football." (October 6).

NIH Consensus Statement. January 21–23, 1997. "Breast Cancer Screening for Women Ages 40–49" 15: 1–35.

Norsigian, Judy. 1992. "The Women's Health Movement in the United States." *WGNRR (Women's Global Network on Reproductive Rights* 39: 9–12.

Norsigian, Judy, and Jane Pincus. 1992. "Organizing for Change: U.S.A." Pp. 699–708 in *The New Our Bodies, Ourselves: A Book by and for Women. Updated and expanded Version for 1990s*, ed. the Boston Women's Health Book Collective. New York: Touchstone.

Norwood, Chris. 1988. "Alarming Rise in Deaths." *Ms.* 17: 65, 67.

———. 1990. "Media Coverage on Women and AIDS: Bias, Negative Imagery, and Exclusion of Women's Experts and Sources." Pp. 5–22 in *The Guide to Resources on Women and AIDS*, ed. the Center for Women Policy Studies. Washington, D.C.: Center for Women Policy Studies.

O'Hanlan, Katherine A. 1995. "Lesbians in Health Research." Pp. 101–104 in *Recruitment and Retention of Women in Clinical Studies*, ed. U.S. Department of Health and Human Services. NIH Publication No. 95-3756.

Olson, Mancur. 1965. *The Logic of Collective Action*. Cambridge, Mass.: Harvard University Press.

Omoto, Allen M., and A. Lauren Crain. 1995. "AIDS Volunteerism: Lesbian and Gay Community-Based Responses to HIV." Pp. 187–209 in *AIDS Identity, and Community: The HIV Epidemic and Lesbians and Gay Men*, ed. Gregory M. Herek and Beverly Greene. Thousand Oaks, Calif.: Sage.

Omoto, Allen M., and Mark Snyder. 1990. "Basic Research in Action: Volunteerism and Society's Response to AIDS." *Personality and Social Psychology Bulletin* 16: 152–65.

Omoto, Allen M., Mark Snyder, and James P. Berghuis. 1993. "The Psychology of Volunteerism: A Conceptual Analysis and a Program of Action Research." Pp. 333–56 in *The Social Psychology of HIV Infection*, ed. J. B. Pryor and G. D. Reeder. Hillsdale, N.J.: Lawrence Erlbaum Associates.

Patterson, James T. 1987. *The Dread Disease: Cancer and Modern American Culture*. Cambridge, Mass.: Harvard University Press.

Patton, Cindy. 1990. *Inventing AIDS*. New York and London: Routledge.

Penelope, Julia. 1990. "The Lesbian Perspective." Pp. 89–108 in *Lesbian Philosophies and Cultures*, ed. Jeffner Allen. Albany, N.Y.: State University of New York Press.

People with AIDS/ARC. 1990. "The Denver Principles." Pp. 239ff. in *Women, AIDS & Activism*, ed. the ACT UP/NY Women and AIDS Book Group. Boston: South End.

Peterson, K. Jean, and Mary Bricker Jenkins. 1996. "Lesbians and the Health Care System." *Journal of Gay and Lesbian Social Services* 5: 33–47.

Posner, Prudence S. 1990. "Introduction." Pp. 3–20 in *Dilemmas of Activism: Class, Community, and the Politics of Local Mobilization*, ed. Joseph M. Kling and Prudence S. Posner. Philadelphia: Temple University Press.

Poullard, Jonathan D., and Anthony R. D'Augelli. 1989. "AIDS Fear and Homophobia among Volunteers in an AIDS Prevention Program." *Journal for Rural Community Psychology* 10: 29–39.

Rachel's Children. 1995. Newsletter, Vol. 1 (June).

Rachel's Children: Fighting for Our Lives. 1995. Newsletter. *Women, Health and the Environment*.

Rainbow News. 1996. Vol. 1.

Rich, Adrienne. 1983. "Compulsory Heterosexuality and Lesbian Existence." Pp. 177–205 in *Powers of Desire: The Politics of Sexuality*, ed. Ann Snitow, Christine Stansell, and Sharon Thompson. New York: Monthly Review Press.

Ries, Lynn A., Barry A. Gloeckler, Benjamin F. Miller, Carol L. Hankey, Angela Harras Kosary, and Brenda K. Edwards, eds. 1994. *SEER Cancer Statistics Review, 1973–1991: Tables and Graphs*. Bethesda, Md.: National Cancer Institute.

Rofes, Eric. 1995. *Reviving the Tribe: Regenerating Gay Men's Sexuality and Culture in the Ongoing Epidemic*. New York: Harrington Park Press.

———. 1990. "Gay Groups vs. AIDS Groups: Averting Civil War in the 1990s." *OUT/LOOK* 2: 8–17.

Rollin, Betty. 1976. *First You Cry*. New York: New American Library.

Rosser, Sue V. 1994. *Women's Health—Missing from U.S. Medicine*. Bloomington and Indianapolis: Indiana University Press.

Rudner, Delaynie. 1995. "The Censored Scar." *Gauntlet* 2: 13–27.

Ruzek, Sheryl Burt. 1978. *The Women's Health Movement: Feminist Alternatives to Medical Control*. New York: Praeger.

Ryan, Barbara. 1992. *Feminism and the Women's Movement: Dynamics of Change in Social Movement, Ideology and Activism*. New York: Routledge.

Sacks, Valerie. 1996. "Women and AIDS: An Analysis of Media Misrepresentations." *Social Science and Medicine* 42: 59–73.

Schable, B., S. Y. Chu, and T. Diaz. 1996. "Characteristics of Women 50 Years of Age of Older with Heterosexually Acquired AIDS." *American Journal of Public Health* 86: 1616–18.

Schneider, Beth E. 1992. "AIDS and Class, Gender, and Race Relations." Pp. 19–43 in *The Social Context of AIDS*, ed. Joan Huber and Beth E. Schneider. Newbury Park, Calif.: Sage.

Schulman, Sarah. 1994. *My American History: Lesbian and Gay Life during the Reagan/Bush Years*. New York: Routledge.

Shapiro, Susan. 1989. "Cancer As a Feminist Issue." *Sojourner* (September).

Shilts, Randy M. 1987. *And the Band Played On: Politics, People and the AIDS Epidemic*. New York: St. Martin's Press.

Siegel, K., D. Karus, and V. H. Raveis. 1997. "Testing and Treatment Behaviour of HIV-Infected Women: White, African-American, Puerto Rican Comparisons." *AIDS Care* 9: 297–309.

Signorile, Michelangelo. 1993. *Queer in America: Sex, the Media, and the Closets of Power*. New York: Random House.

Snitow, Ann, Christine Stansell, and Sharon Thompson, eds. 1983. *Powers of Desire: The Politics of Sexuality*. New York: Monthly Review Press.

Snow, David A., Louis A. Zurcher, and Sheldon Ekland-Olson. 1980. "Social Networks and Social Movements: A Microstructural Approach to Differential Recruitment." *American Sociological Review* 45: 787–801.

Snyder, Mark, and Allen M. Omoto. 1992. "Volunteerism and Society's Response to the HIV Epidemic." *Current Directions in Psychological Science* 3: 113–16.

Solomon, Alisa. 1991. "The Politics of Breast Cancer." *Village Voice* (May 14): 22–27.

Spelman, Elizabeth V. 1988. *Inessential Woman: Problems of Exclusion in Feminist Thought*. Boston: Beacon Press.

Stan, Adele M., ed. 1995. *Debating Sexual Correctness: Pornography, Sexual Harassment, Date Rape, and the Politics of Sexual Equality*. New York: Delta.

Stein, Arlene. 1995. "Sisters and Queers: The Decentering of Lesbian Feminism." Pp. 133–53 in *Cultural Politics and Social Movements*, ed. Marcy Darnovsky, Barbara Epstein, and Richard Flacks. Philadelphia: Temple University Press.

Steingraber, Sandra. 1993. " 'If I Live to be 90 Still Wanting to Say Something': My Search for Rachel Carson." Pp. 181–200 in *Confronting Cancer, Constructing Change: New Perspectives on Women and Cancer*, ed. Midge Stocker. Chicago, Ill.: Third Side Press.

Stevens, Patricia E. 1993. "Lesbians and HIV: Clinical, Research, and Policy Issues." *American Journal of Orthopsychiatry* 63: 289–94.

Stoller, Nancy. 1995a. "Lesbian Involvement in the AIDS Epidemic: Changing Roles and Generational Differences." Pp. 270–285 in *Women Resisting AIDS: Feminist Strategies of Empowerment*, ed. Beth E. Schneider and Nancy E. Stoller. Philadelphia: Temple University Press.

———. 1995b. "Racial Prescriptions for Sexual Permissions: Ideological Messages in AIDS Prevention Materials." Presented at *Annual Meeting of the American Sociological Association*, August 19–23. Washington, D.C.

Szaz, Andrew. 1994. *EcoPopulism: Toxic Waste and the Movement for Environmental Justice*. Minneapolis: University of Minnesota Press.

Tallen, Bette S. 1990. "How Inclusive Is Feminist Theory? Questions for Lesbians?" Pp. 241–57 in *Lesbian Philosophies and Cultures*, ed. Jeffner Allen. Albany, N.Y.: State University of New York Press.

Tarrow, Sidney. 1994. *Power in Movement: Social Movements, Collective Action and Politics*. New York: Cambridge University Press.

Trippet, Susan E., and Joyce Bain. 1993. "Physical Health Problems and Concerns of Lesbians." *Women and Health* 20: 59–70.

US TOO. 1998a. *Hot Sheet* (March).

———. 1998b. "Organization Introduction." website: www.ustoo.com.

Vaid, Urvashi. 1995. *Virtual Equality: The Mainstreaming of Gay and Lesbian Liberation*. New York: Anchor Books.

Ward, Debbie. 1995. "Women and Health Care." Pp. 111–24 in *Women's Health Care: A Comprehensive Handbook*, ed. Catherine Ingram Fogel and Nancy Fugate Woods. Thousand Oaks, Calif.: Sage.

Weinberg, George. 1972. *Society and the Healthy Homosexual*. Boston: Alyson.

Whittier, Nancy. 1995. *Feminist Generations: The Persistence of the Radical Women's Movement*. Philadelphia: Temple University Press.

Winnow, Jackie. 1991. "Lesbians Evolving Health Care: Our Lives Depend on It." Pp. 23–35 in *Cancer as a Women's Issue: Scratching the Surface*, ed. Midge Stocker. Chicago, Ill.: Third Side Press.

———. 1993. "The Politics of Cancer." Pp. 153–63 in *Confronting Cancer, Constructing Change: New Perspectives on Women and Cancer*, ed. Midge Stocker. Chicago, Ill.: Third Side Press.

Winslow, Cindy. 1991. "A Letter to My Doctor." Pp. 129–36 in *One in Three: Women with Cancer Confront an Epidemic*, ed. Judith Brady. Pittsburgh and San Francisco: Cleis Press.

Women and AIDS Coalition. 1992. "Women and AIDS Coalition 1993 Mission and Priorities." Pp. 3–20 in *The Guide to Resources on Women and AIDS*, ed. the Center for Women Policy Studies. Washington, D.C.: Center for Women Policy Studies.

Women's Community Cancer Project. 1993. "Demands to the NCI and the U.S. Government." Pp. 261–63 in *Confronting Cancer, Constructing Change: New Perspectives on Women and Cancer*, ed. Midge Stocker. Chicago, Ill.: Third Side Press.

Women's Environment & Development Organization and Greenpeace. 1994. "We Are Rachel's Children." P. 4 in *Breast Cancer Action*. Newsletter.

Yockey, Cynthia. 1987. "AIDS: Sidetracking Feminism. A Conversation with Sonia Johnson." *Lambda Risking Book Report* 1: 1, 5.

Young, Rebecca M. 1997. *HIV/AIDS and Women Who Have Sex with Women*. Presentation to the Institute of Medicine Workshop on Lesbian Health Research Priorities. Georgetown University Conference Center, Washington, D.C., October 6–7.

Zimmerman, Mary K. 1987. "The Women's Health Movement: A Critique of Medical Enterprise and the Position of Women." Pp. 442–72 in *Analyzing Gender: A Handbook of Social Science Research*, ed. Myra Marx Ferree and Beth B. Hess. Newbury Park, Calif.: Sage.

Index